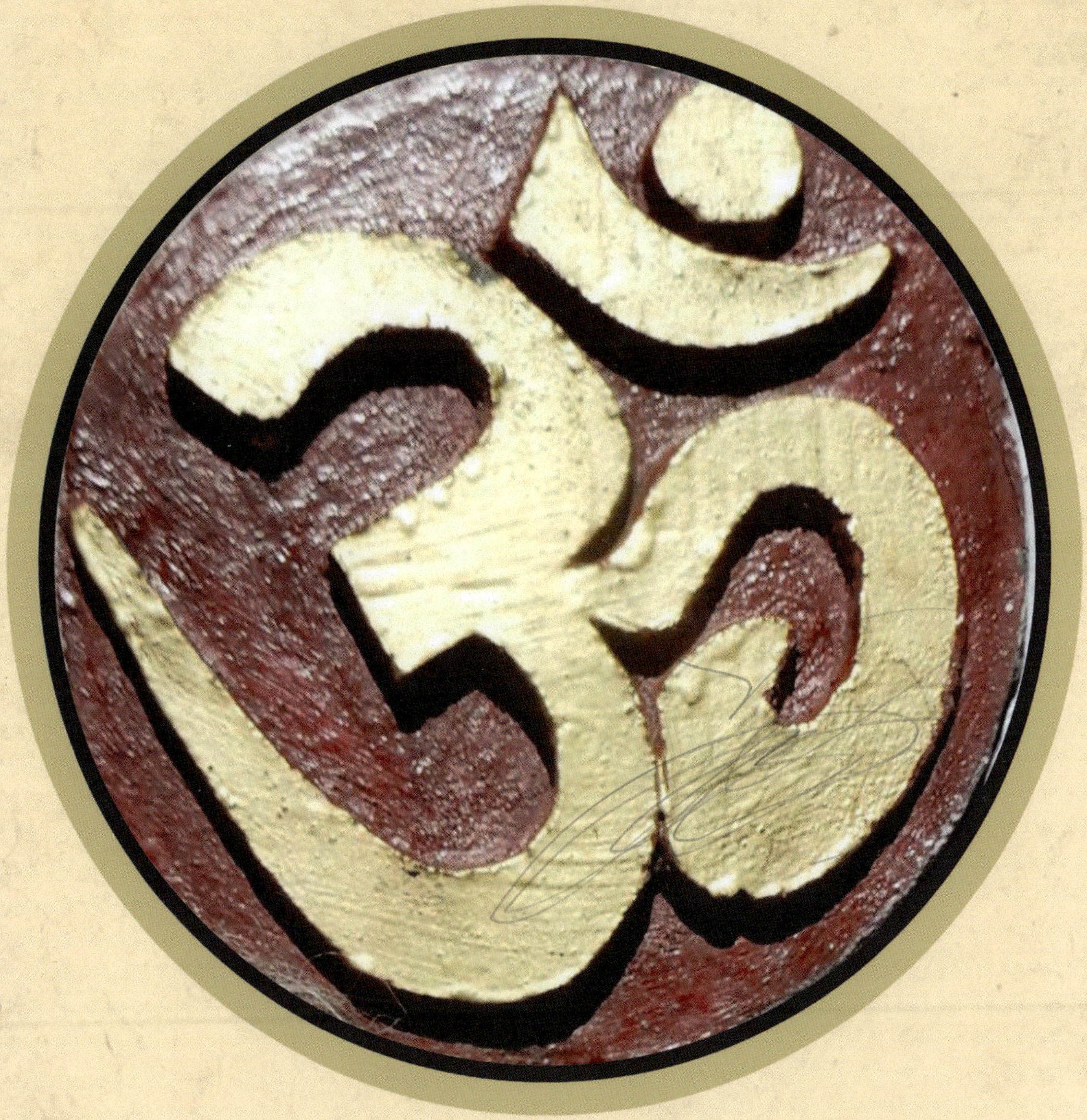

ISBN 978-0-2285-0733-8

Author: Phoebe Bowman (www.phoebewriting.com)
Artwork and Design: Nicola North Graphic Design (www.nicolanorthart.ca)
Printed and Bound by First Choice Books in Victoria, British Columbia, Canada

Available at Amazon.ca: Kindle Store

With gratitude to Mr. Praveen Juyal of Whoopee Holidays India for organizing the amazing trip itinerary and to Mr. Santosh Sharma, my extraordinary guide.

A WIDOW'S JOURNEY TO THE LAND OF THE GODS

UTTARAKHAND, INDIA

A 26-day journey to Uttarakhand, India in the year 2019, captured in daily journal description, my photos and poetry, and embedded with memories of my husband as I also travel through the process of grief.

PHOEBE BOWMAN

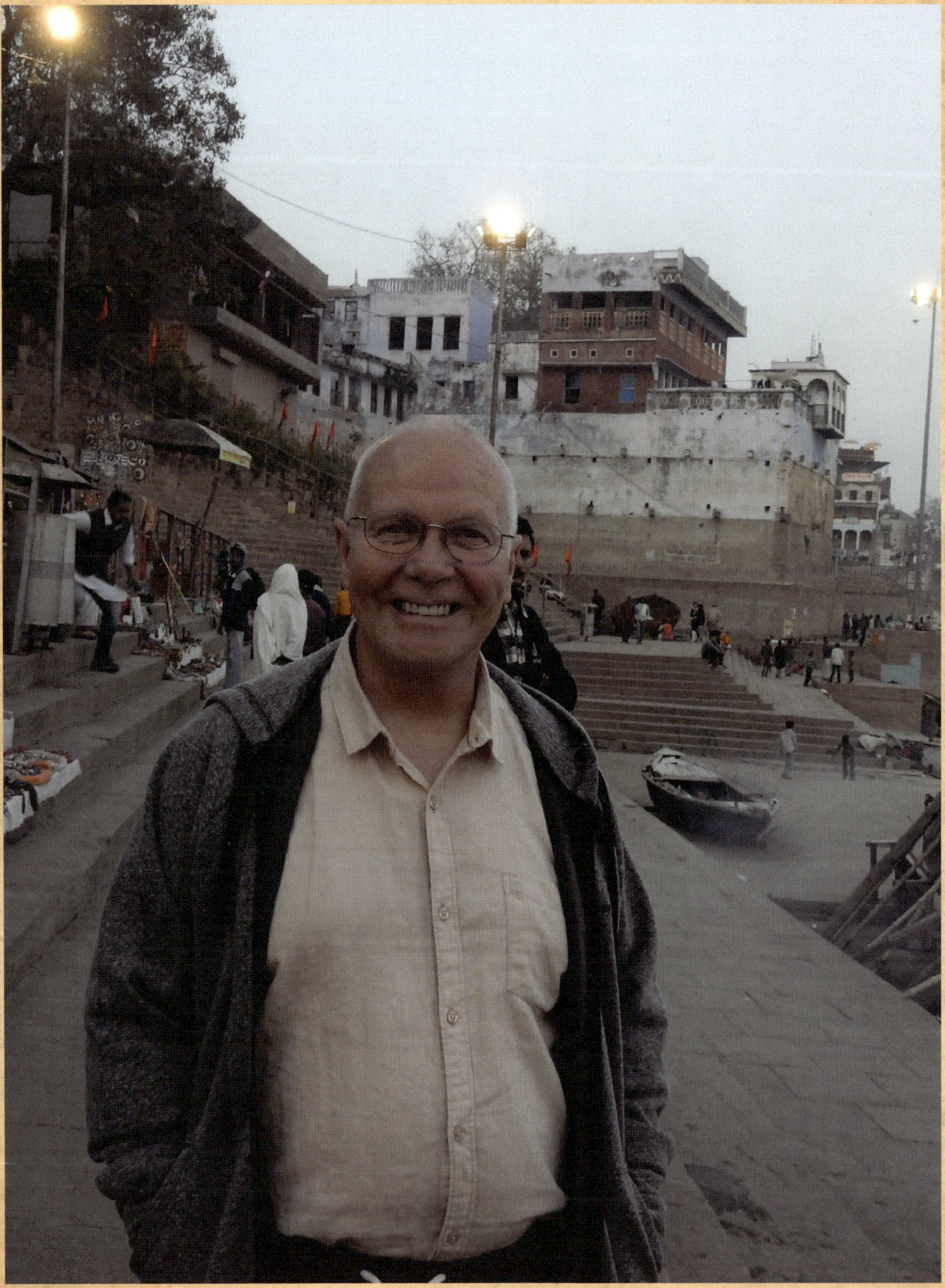

DEDICATION

This book is dedicated to my beloved husband of forty years, Kelly Ross Bowman.

In February of 2017, Kelly and I travelled to the incredible country of India as a last big adventure together. At the time, Kelly knew he was dying from metastatic prostate cancer. But he had no pain and an indomitable spirit and he went to India full throttle, feeling and experiencing at the highest level. He ate the hottest chilis, observed street people like local electricians and fishermen and got right into conversation with them about what they were doing and how they lived their lives. He had his head shaved bald with a straight edged razor on the banks of the Ganges River in Varanasi.

Kelly passed away one year later in the comfort of the home he had built in the middle of a five-acre forest. My journey of grief began at his last breath. And yet his warm spirit remains strongly within me, guiding me and encouraging me to continue to live with wonder, joy and adventure.

I will always love you, darling.

You are my forever.

My Journey Begins

I decided to go to India one year after my husband, Kelly, passed away. It would be my third time to visit. The first time I visited was in 2015 when I had the wonderful good fortune for two weeks on my own to connect with a very professional travel organizer, Mr. Praveen Juyal, and experienced travel guide, Mr. Santosh Sharma. I enjoyed all the sights, the temples, and the food. From that experience, I told Kelly that he must see India. We had seen so many other areas of the world together: Cambodia, China, Vietnam, South Africa and Zimbabwe. He was a classic intrepid traveler. When he knew he had not much time left to live, I asked again, and he said yes, I will go to India, and he said "I want to be amazed." I am happy to say I amazed him with that trip in 2017 – the Taj Mahal, toy train to Shimla, elephant bath with Kelly on top to receive the splash, Iskon Krishna temple and all the music and chanting, hair shave at the Ganges River in Varanasi and the powerful Aarti ceremony by the water's edge, canal rides in Kerala, and sitting with the fishermen on the banks of the South Arabian Sea. So now I have returned to India in February of 2019 to find some comfort as a widow and to somehow challenge myself as I carry on in this world without my husband of forty years. I want to rekindle my inner soul that has been dimmed through deep sorrow, on this 26-day journey through Uttarakhand, India, otherwise mystically known as Land of the Gods, Dev Bhoomi.

I endure the 14-hour flight from Vancouver to Hong Kong, the 6-hour layover in Hong Kong, and the final 5-hour flight from Hong Kong to New Delhi. Once in New Delhi and going through Indian Customs and Immigration, I realize I am moving a lot slower and my one foot is sore; I wonder if I can keep travelling anymore. I wonder now if I can travel alone as an aging female with no partner either with me or even waiting at home to help me if needed.

As the taxi cab drives me in the late-night darkness of New Delhi towards my hotel, through the city that does not sleep, my energy returns. It is 10 pm and all the city is still in motion with the honking of the cars, the roadside barber shops, and the tiny brightly-lit dhaba roadside cafes in full swing for night-time customers. A tall, slim, professional looking man is striding solo and with graceful posture alongside the busy highway leading to the airport; he is right next to the racing cars and looking completely calm. I remember again the excitement of India where individuals are energized by the constant abiding with their Gods and Goddesses.

Day 1

New Delhi

I wake up refreshed and indulge as usual in a delicious Indian-style breakfast at my Justa hotel. I always miss my Indian food when I go back home. I think the spicing is so healthy for good body function. I have brought my camera but I have no desire to take pictures in the old way of taking thousands and then trimming them back when I get home. My creative energy is lacking or at a standstill now. I think that if I take so many pictures – who will I share them with? Santosh, my wonderful guide from the last two trips, meets me at 10 am in the hotel lobby. Kelly and Santosh became good friends on the last trip and enjoyed many good cups of chai and conversation. Santosh gives his condolences to me and I thank him but as is so often for me, I keep my grief to myself for private moments. Santosh seems to understand that on this trip, I need a lot of quiet time. He says he will take me to places in the city that I have not been to before.

We start by going to a beautiful Shiva temple. He says in the car that going there will be good energy to start the trip. I suddenly feel yes, that is exactly the right way to think, use positive energy and vibration for this trip to the Land of the Gods. I realize that this trip has a deeper purpose and a life of its own, and that I am a traveler destined for a journey that is somehow beyond my understanding.

Inside this beautiful temple, we stand in front of Shiva and Parvati, God and Goddess, and then Goddess Durga and Lord Hanuman. As I stand beside the Linga for Shiva, a beautiful spiritual Indian woman in her 30's gifts me her small copper bowl of water to wash over the Linga. I am always so lucky on my travels to meet the mystics. We are fellow journeyers and we recognize each other on the path. I receive blessings from the attendant Hindu priests, receiving, and then giving back flowers – marigolds and roses.

At the end of the day, Santosh and I go to Balbin's tomb, in a not-so-visited park near an archaeological dig, where more old remnants of ancient life are being uncovered. Kelly would have loved the stonework. It was exactly what he did on our property. Stone lasts forever. He always knew that.

Day 2

New Delhi

Today begins with another beautiful breakfast like yesterday's but also the cook makes me a potato dosa under the excellent supervision of the manager, Mr. Jaspal Bisht, who runs the Justa hotel like a 5-star maître de. Then it is off to my Naadi astrologer, Mr. Thanapal Kanagaraj. I sit in a small waiting room of ten chairs. When he is ready, we first discuss my booklet he had made for me four years ago. This time, he tells me that I will build a house of blessing between the ages of 68 and 70 years old. I will continue to work on my astrology business and on my energy work such that at the age of 70, people will come to me for blessings. He talks about how closely Kelly and I are connected and that thoughts of Kelly will come to me during the day and also in my dreams. He tells me that because of my deep spiritual practice and prayers, I have added 25 to 30 years onto Kelly's life. My prayers continue for him daily and he will have complete peace and happiness. We look at my Tamil Nadu chart and Mr. Kanagaraj explains that there are 27 stars and my star Aswini was the first star. And that my Moon is in my first house so the first star and first moon. He explains that life's ups and downs are like night and day; they are each rhythmic to each other. I remember in Kelly's spiritual reading after his passing, that where he is now has no day or night and that you don't need sleep because you always have energy.

After seeing my astrologer, Santosh and the driver take me to the Hanuman temple which I had visited twice before in previous trips, but there is a long line-up as it is Tuesday, one of the special worship days of Lord Hanuman, and I say no, let's go for lunch. I know I will return at another time. We drive to an amazing South Indian style lunch canteen in a ritzy area of government political offices. We share a table with a son and mother from Kerala and it is nice in conversation with them to remember the beautiful visit Kelly and I had to that gorgeous southern state two years previous. Our lunch is thali style which here is eight small metal bowls of various items like rice, dahl, curried potatoes and peas, carrots with ginger, coconut dessert and papadam, and so delicious.

Finally, Santosh and I go to a coffee shop called "Café Turtle" set two floors up in an old building with a funky bookstore. I order an iced Americano with tasty espresso and no cream or sugar. The time leisurely goes by and I write a poem on the spot. On the wall above me is a fascinating picture of an American Cherokee First Nations man sitting on the grass with a long pipe, and looking serenely out before him, which in this case is over all of us in this New Delhi coffee shop.

The Spirit Soars in Quiet Flight

The spirit soars in quiet flight
The soul free from the body
But still connected to all things
With the thread of love

It is easy to see the mountains
The crags and crevices
It is easy to spot the flowers

My heart connects to the one I love
Who is soaring while I sit
Enjoying my Americano over ice

Day 3

Train from Delhi to Kathgodam, drive from Kathgodam to Kausani

The journey this morning starts early, leaving on the train from New Delhi main rail station at 6:15 am. I am used to this bustling, noisy train station as this is now my third time here. I guess I look experienced as no-one bothers me for carrying my bag. It is also clear I am with my Indian guide, Santosh, who expertly leads me to the right platform. We are in 1st class and everything is calm, clean and orderly. I notice a very elderly woman lying on her back across a long, cushioned seat; her eyes are wide open just staring and she is lying so still she looks frozen in place. But she has family around her and tending to her. I pass her once again as I return to my seat after getting up to stretch my legs, and my eyes lock with her wide-open eyes and her eyes are like saucers and fully in her moment of dying and full knowledge of that. After the long train journey, when we are waiting for the car and driver, I see her in a wheelchair, thin and old, surrounded by a loving family who are taking her home to die. I go over and touch her shoulder and we lock eyes once again and I stare with respect and love into her eyes and say “Goodbye, Momma”. It is a powerful intersection of lives, and I think about my own spiritual journey as a widow and how she must have gone through the same. And now, she is one step ahead of me, and I will go through the same as her at some point and remember her at that time.

Dev Bhoomi, Land of the Gods. I feel that energy immediately upon the start of our drive up through high mountain passes on long narrow roads with many forks. Our expert driver, Mr. Gajendra, proceeds for hours to navigate oncoming cars, motorcycles, school children and dogs. A fork comes and the driver turns and in we go to a whole new mountain pass. We are surrounded by rolling mountains like the multiple sand piles that are left after a tidal ocean recedes. Our driver, called Gajendra after the God Ganesh, points out the higher range of snow-capped Himalayas in the far distance. We are merely in the foothills. On and on, we drive. The local people are strong and fit, full of the energy of the sweet mountain air and the vigour that comes from walking and working on steep mountain slopes. On the way, we stop at a local dhaba which has a wonderful patio set on a slope. In the luxuriant full sun, we eat wild rice mixed with white rice, curry with cheese, and dahl with naan. My lunch is always my supper too, so I eat well. We reach the Heritage Resort hotel at dusk.

The first thing I do when I enter my room is to put on the portable electric heater. Up in the higher elevations, very few hotels have central heating. Suddenly the lights and the heater go out and I think it is Kelly! His words to me in the spiritual reading were "I want you to travel. I will be going with you" I request an extra quilt, the lights come back on and into bed I go at 7 pm with my hat, sweater, coat and socks. I actually sleep very well. Kelly was always impressed with how fast I could fall asleep and how soundly I sleep. I think it is the result of a peaceful mind.

I wake at 4 am and step outside onto the balcony. My room may be stone-cold but it has a spectacular view of the distant Himalayan high mountains. I remember again my visit to my Naadi astrologer, Mr. Kanagaraj. I had asked him more about my star which is Aswini. It is the first of 27 stars. Does this mean there are 27 solar systems? I must ask him that on the last Sunday before I leave when I have another visit planned. Perhaps the spiritual lesson on this trip is to experience a sense of the different star systems and incorporate them into my astrology practice and into my own sense of soul knowledge. I reflect a lot also on what Mr. Kanagaraj said about Kelly dying 25 to 30 years earlier except for my deep spiritual practice and devotion to him. Before his terminal illness, Kelly lived a wonderful life on our country acreage. He had a seventeen-year project of building a house, putting in a series of rustic buildings called Whoville and setting down, using rock from our own property, multiple beautiful stone pathways, especially down to the creek running through our acreage. My astrologer guide said Kelly is now working on soul issues that come from karmic patterning. I have entered into a gift of eight months of chanting by a temple priest to dissolve those patterns. The astrologer said that Kelly had the abilities of being a mechanical engineer, and I personally had seen that ability many times. But his birth family/karmic patterning destroyed the pathway necessary to achieve this high goal. Now my sincere and intense prayer for him is for him to have the clarity and peace of mind to proceed with his engineering gift whether in his present spiritual circumstance or again on earth in a circumstance where he can be supported and trained for this, thrive and become respected and acknowledged.

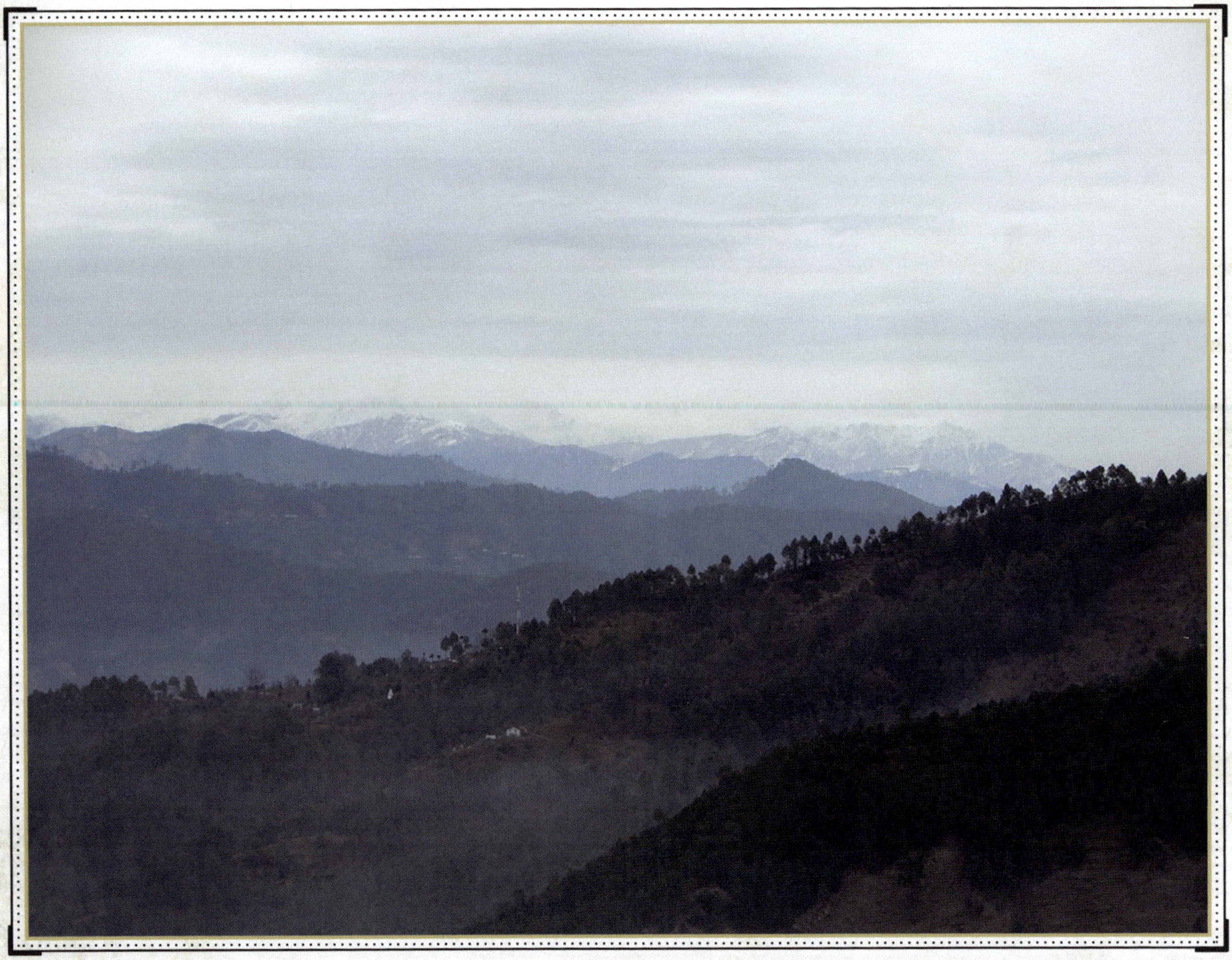

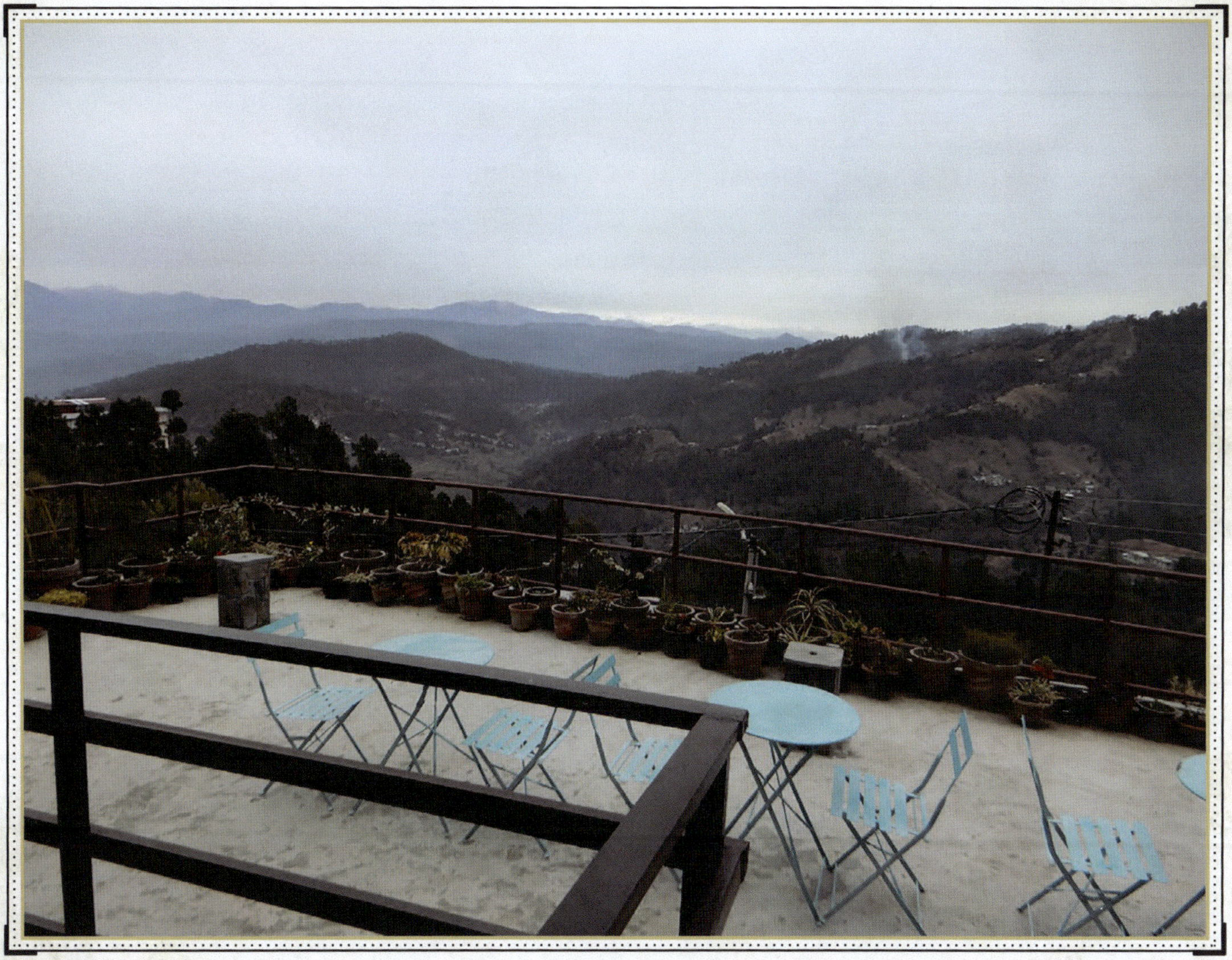

Day 4

(full day in Kausani)

Last night, I dreamt of a big cat; I think it was a leopard. I was on an escalator in a department store, going up, and I saw that the leopard had escaped and was roaming freely throughout the store. I was aware but not worried and knew I should just act naturally with it. I am starting to sense some of the powers of the Himalayas in animal form. Today is beautiful and mystical. Santosh and Gajendra pick me up at 10 am after my delicious breakfast of stuffed potato paratha, masala omelette, and white coffee (coffee with steamed milk and a little sugar.) We amble our way for 4 km along a quiet narrow road with little traffic in a seemingly out-of-the-way country area. We descend a bit and then a picturesque small town, Baijnath, comes into view. We pass one exquisite house with an ornate orange wrought-iron fence. Other houses are brightly colored in greens and pinks. We make our way into the town centre and then slightly outside of it to an old Shiva temple, Baijnath temple, built in the early 1200's and now a protected site. It is still an active temple and, on this site, God Shiva and his Goddess Parvati came to visit. This is a very special place in spirit energy. We walk down a long walkway and on entering the temple grounds, as usual, remove our shoes. The temple is a collection of old stone small shrines. We each ring the large ornate bell to announce our arrival to the Gods.

The temple is set next to a small lake and this alone creates its beauty as water has memory, and the memory is of a God and a Goddess. Inside the Parvati shrine, Santosh shows me the rituals of prayer and offering. The priest at the small door has already placed the red (female) and white (male) bindi powders on my 3rd eye area. Parvati's beautiful statue stands in front of us with a Shiva Linga close by in front of her. To honour them both, we are each given a small copper pot and we make our way to the small lake where we fill our small pots with water, after stepping down stone steps to the lake. We return to the shrine, and carefully pour the water over the top of the Linga with the water spreading over its sides. Santosh explains that devotees will also offer beautiful flowers such as marigolds.

We step back outside from the darker stone-walled space into the small courtyard. A priest is performing a puja ceremony for an older couple and their son, with all of them on an upraised platform. There is burning incense on a small fire and the priest's chanting fills the air. And then, because I am used to looking into the sky so that I can observe the formation of clouds, I see that the clouds above us have an unusual energy. I can see small edges of colour of a very light pink and turquoise blue. And then I see that the clouds also have the pattern of a circle with a clear space in the middle. I perceive this to be the eye of Shiva watching us as our energy bodies walk around the temple.

It is a special omen as we enter deeper into this Kingdom. We put our shoes back on and stand a short while under a very old tree. We walk back up the long walkway where one old man with gnarled and amputated finger ends sits quietly at the side of the walkway. I give him alms and, as I put my hands over his to send him loving energy, he chants a Shiva prayer.

Now it is chai time, and we travel along the road back out. We find a small shop for novelty items and order a chai which is delivered to us in small silver cups, steaming hot and delicious. We join a lone man who has a large tree root and stump burning at low ebb. He is sitting on a log with a tarp overtop to keep out the occasional burst of rain. He has a kettle of water at a low boil for the needs of the small store across the street from which we had ordered the chai. We drink the hot chai next to this glowing fire with smoke shifting in direction. How many hundreds of times had Kelly and I done exactly this, with wood and root from our own property down in the small "village" of hand-hewn huts built by Kelly on our property, called "Whoville".

It is too early to stop for the day so on we go to a Gandhi ashram set higher up above the main town of Kausani. The ashram has a magnificent view of the entire valley with the higher Himalayas set majestically behind. We take pictures of the Gandhi statue and talk of his life and great service to the country which through his efforts became free and independent again after 300 years of British rule. On our way back to the hotel, I stop at a shawl shop. I have learned there is a very large cottage industry here of knitted goods such as sweaters and blankets, hats and gloves. I purchase two brightly colored sweaters, one bright green and one lavender pink. I think I will come back the next day and get a hat and maybe shawl for over my coat. We are not yet at the coldest destinations on this trip and I have packed too lightly.

Finally, we drive back to my hotel and I invite Santosh and Gajendra to lunch at the restaurant. The breakfast was delicious so I know lunch will be too. It does not disappoint with a very organic, local dahl with onion and mushroom base, mustard raita which is a specialty local dish, a whole grain naan, a mushroom curry dish, and finally a vegetarian biryani rice dish. Simply exquisite. The food is one of the reasons I always come back to India. I return to my room with a steaming cup of fresh ginger-spiced chai and sit outside for about an hour just enjoying the sounds of car horns, birds and dogs, and many school children laughing and chattering as they walk home. I watch the clouds play over the valley, set against the distant but present tallest Himalaya peaks.

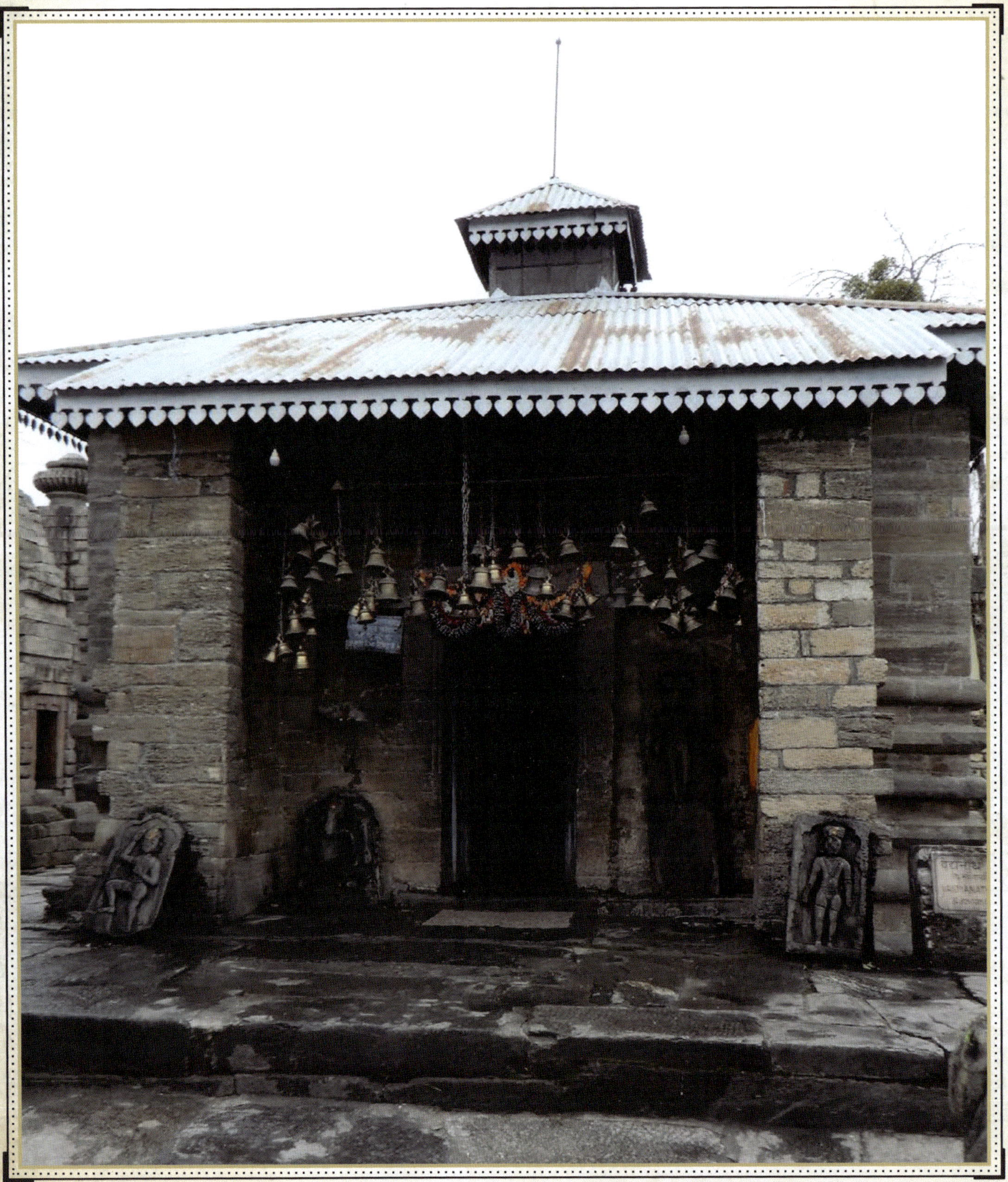

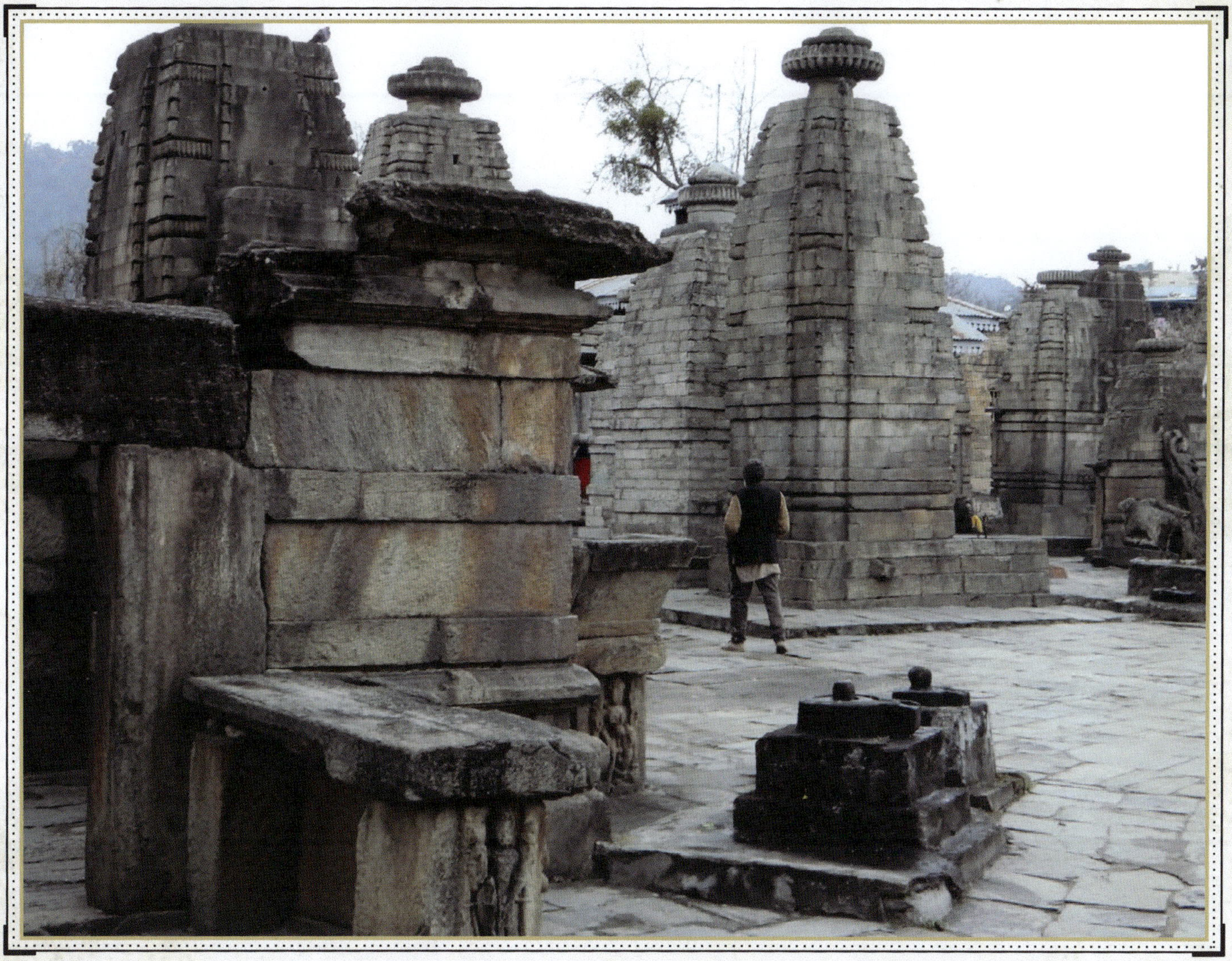

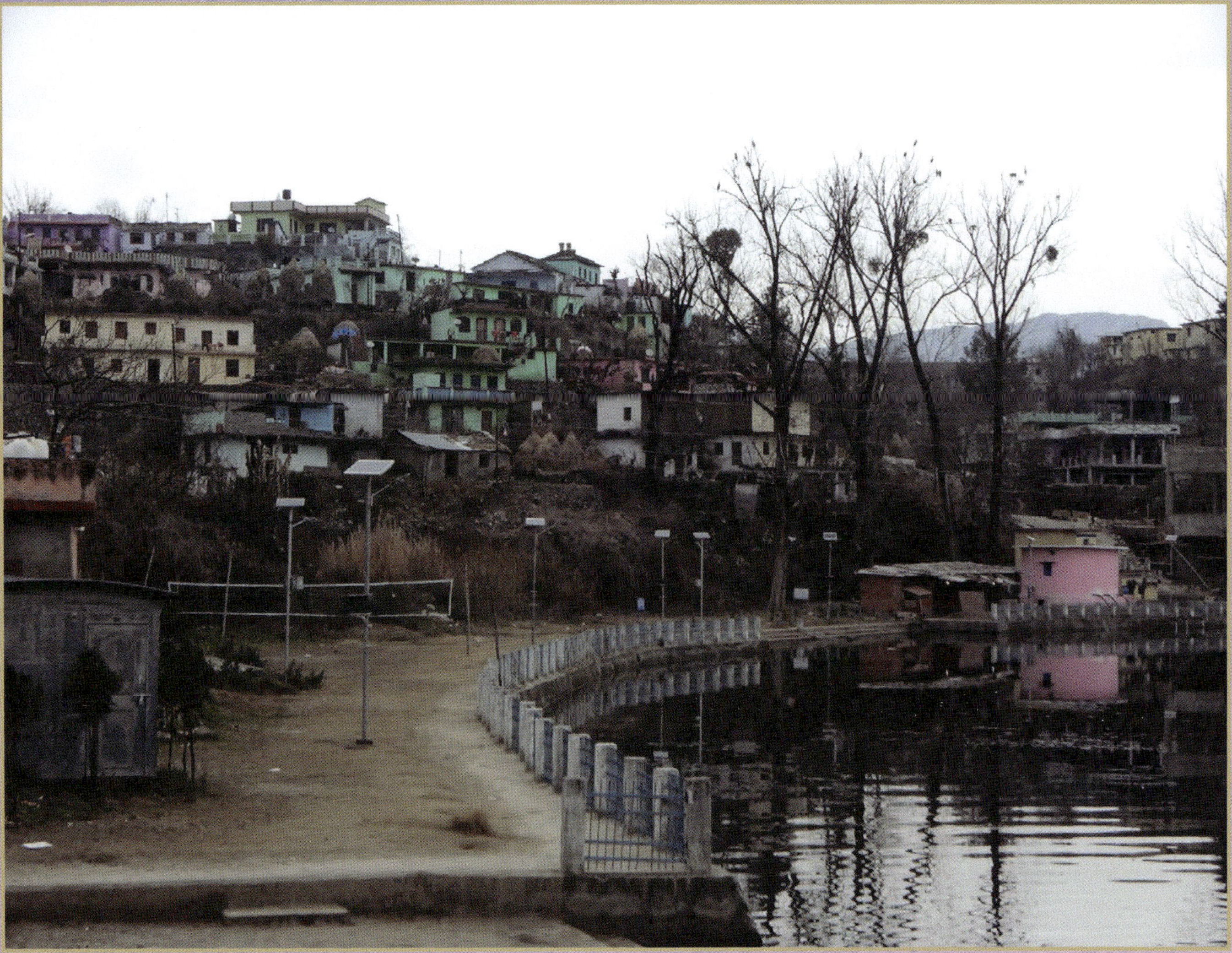

The Eye of Shiva

Today, I was blessed with the Eye of Shiva
He is sitting in these hills
A wild man sometimes tamed with the heart of Parvati
But always running loose and powerful

Today, I was blessed with the Eye of Shiva
The clouds above the Temple
Suddenly tinted with pink and purple
Forming into a circle
At the centre of which lies the Eye
He is watching us, observing us
These three spiritual seekers on his Temple grounds

Today, I was blessed with the Eye of Shiva
Who watched as I held the gnarled hands of an old man
Who has himself been blessed many times by Shiva
Although you would not know it seeing his frozen fingers
But his heart is as wild as Shiva's
And they play together after dark

Last night, I dreamt of a beautiful leopard
Roaming free where I walked
And as I write this, the rain starts on the roof

The Eye is watching
The leopard heart is waiting
I am open to the energy of the Gods
My eye is watching too

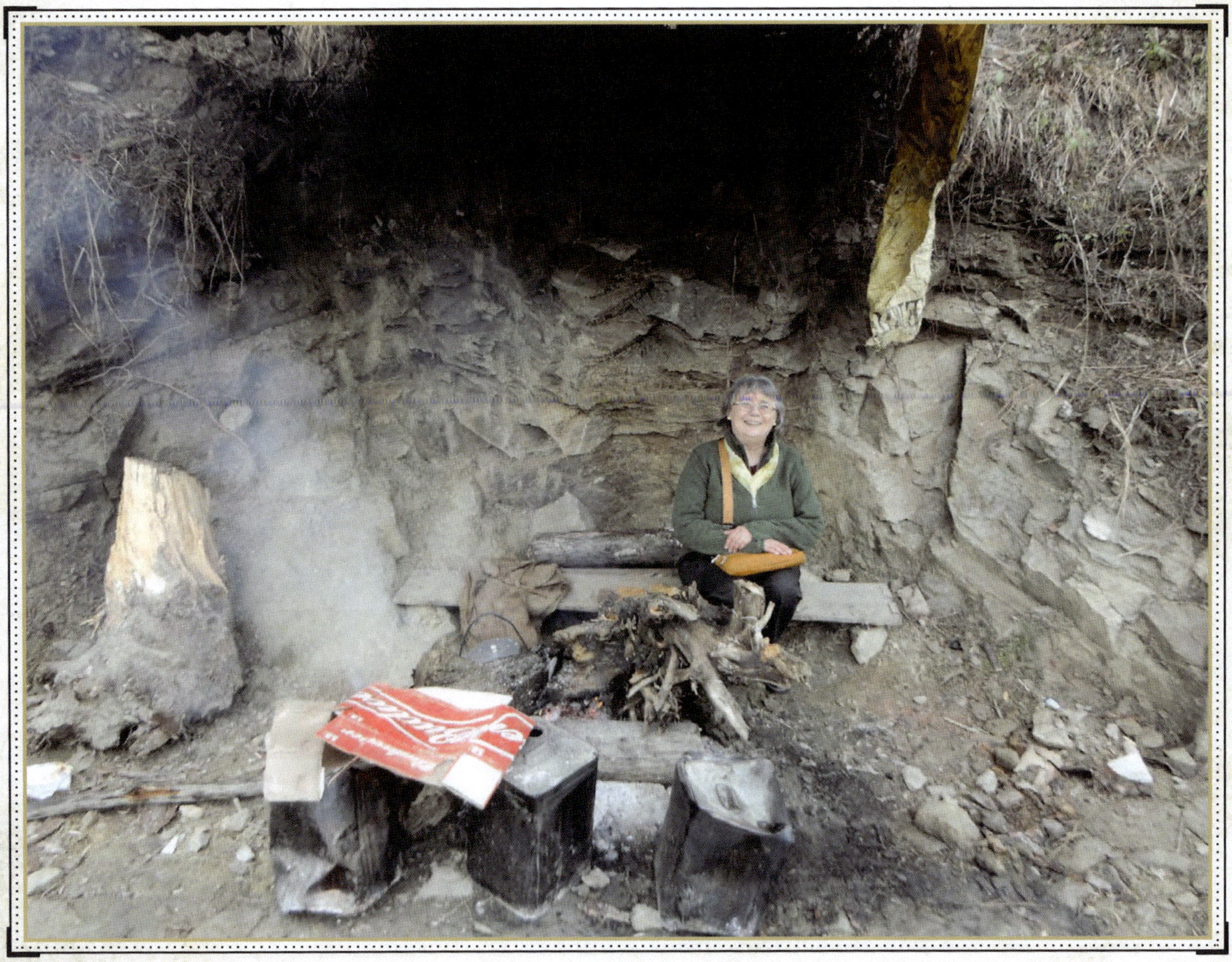

Day 5

(Kausani to Ranikhet)

Another delicious breakfast with potato-stuffed paratha, masala omelette, cut-up apple, and white coffee. Santosh meets me at 10 am and tells me he has dreamt of God, of Lord Shiva. How amazing and special is that. Yes, the Shiva temple here is powerful with a strong mystic presence. I mention I would like to stop again at the Kausani woollen fixed-price shop and there I pick up a pink woollen hat, a beautiful green and black woven shawl and woollen socks to be used at night on the sometimes cold, floor tiles. On we go, with the day being spent on the road going through remote country village areas. The valleys are filled with mustard yellow plots intermixed with green shrubs. Occasionally, the sun comes out warmly and it feels here like perfection; happy people in a happy place surrounded by bush pine forests. We descend into one valley and then rise up the side of another mountain. We are changing locations through this rolling network of Himalayan mountains.

We reach Ranikhet which is very much a military town with a large military base. There is also a busy bus station with buses leaving to all areas of India. The room in the Woods Villa Resort has a magnificent view of the Himalayas and, in the evening, I watch the rain clouds come and go in the far distance against the backdrop of a mountain so magnificent with grandeur and snow, it is like Mount Everest. It makes me realize how great an endeavour it was and is for the climbers of these vastly tall mountains. In the late morning, we visit Jhula Devi, an 8th century temple, as our outing for the day. This temple is a female Goddess temple. On this site, a man received a vision from the Goddess Durga to dig on the top of this mountain and there he found a statue of the Goddess. The vision also told him to build a temple. In the old days of man-eating tigers, once the temple was built, even the tigers respected the power of the area and left it alone.

The temple is closed but we circumambulate the temple and see hundreds of brass bells of all sizes cascading from the fence. The bells are brought to the temple as gifts to the Goddess for her blessing. Just outside the temple as we leave, we see a small hut that sells coconut for offerings and we order chai. The family is friendly and I sit with the 100-year-old matriarch and have a picture taken with her. I am back to the hotel for a light lunch and then retire into the coldness of night. It is so cold I use two quilts, wrapping myself in them like a sleeping bag. It is a two-hat night, it is so cold. But I fall asleep with the single heater set on a table aimed right at me.

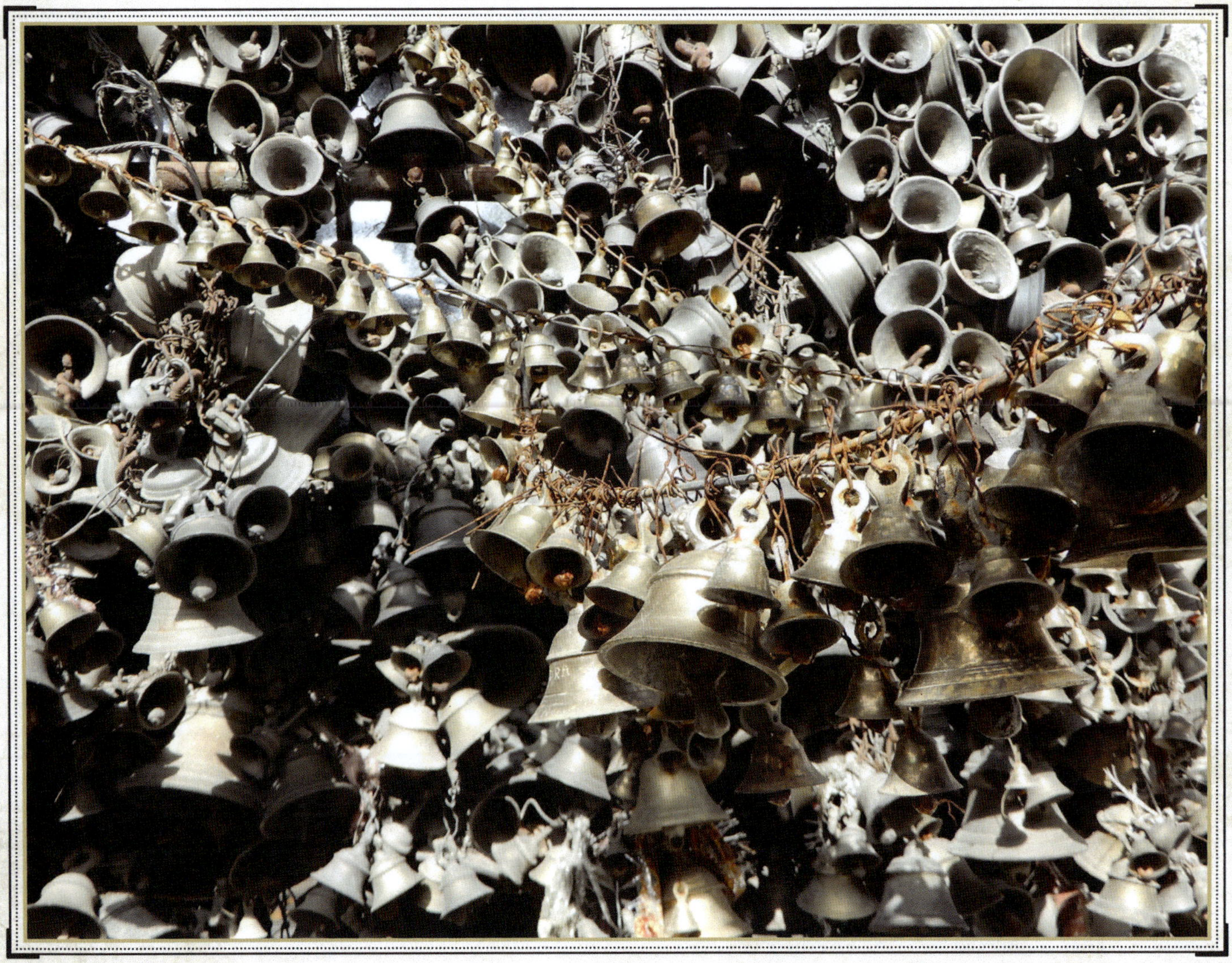

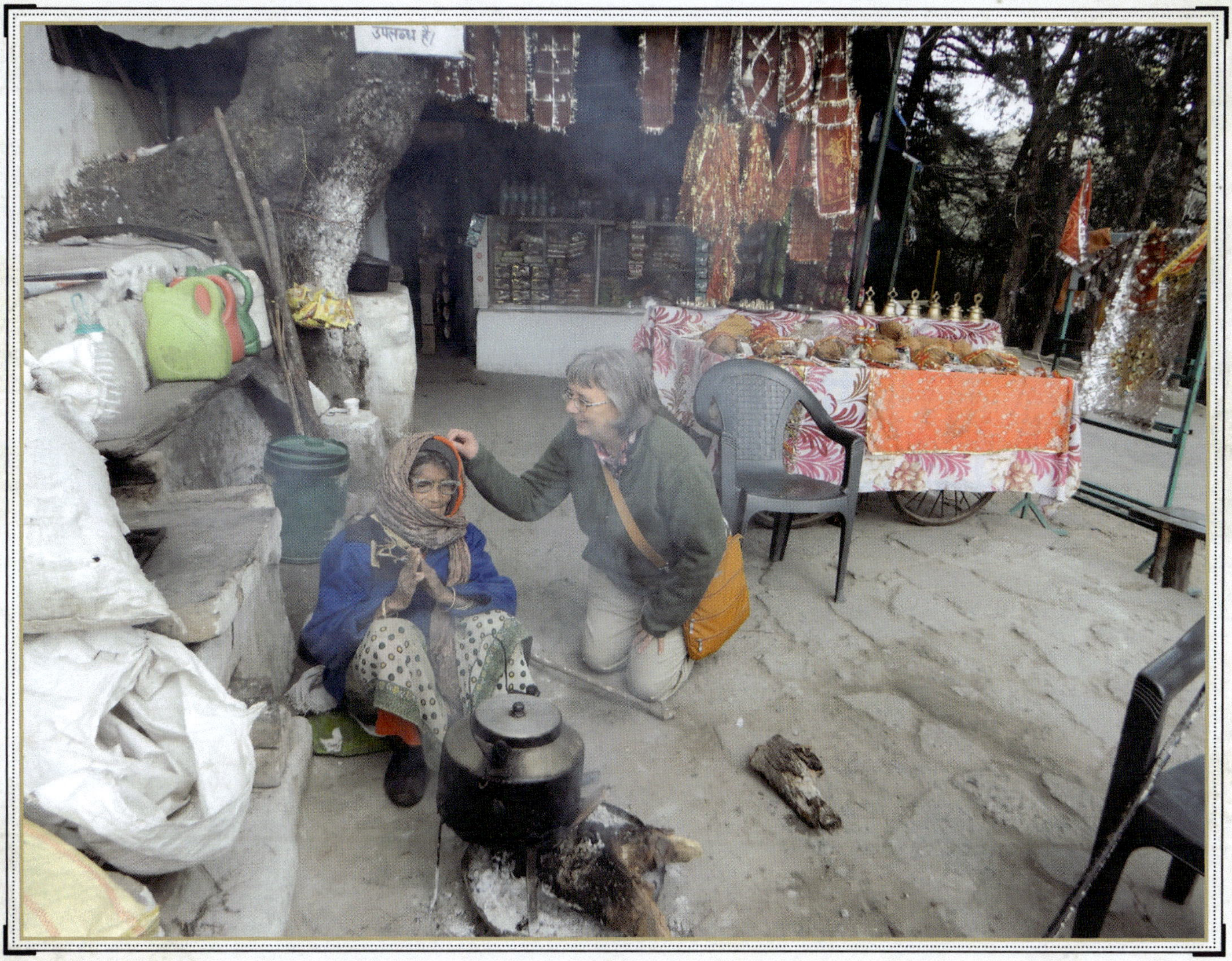
उपलब्ध है।

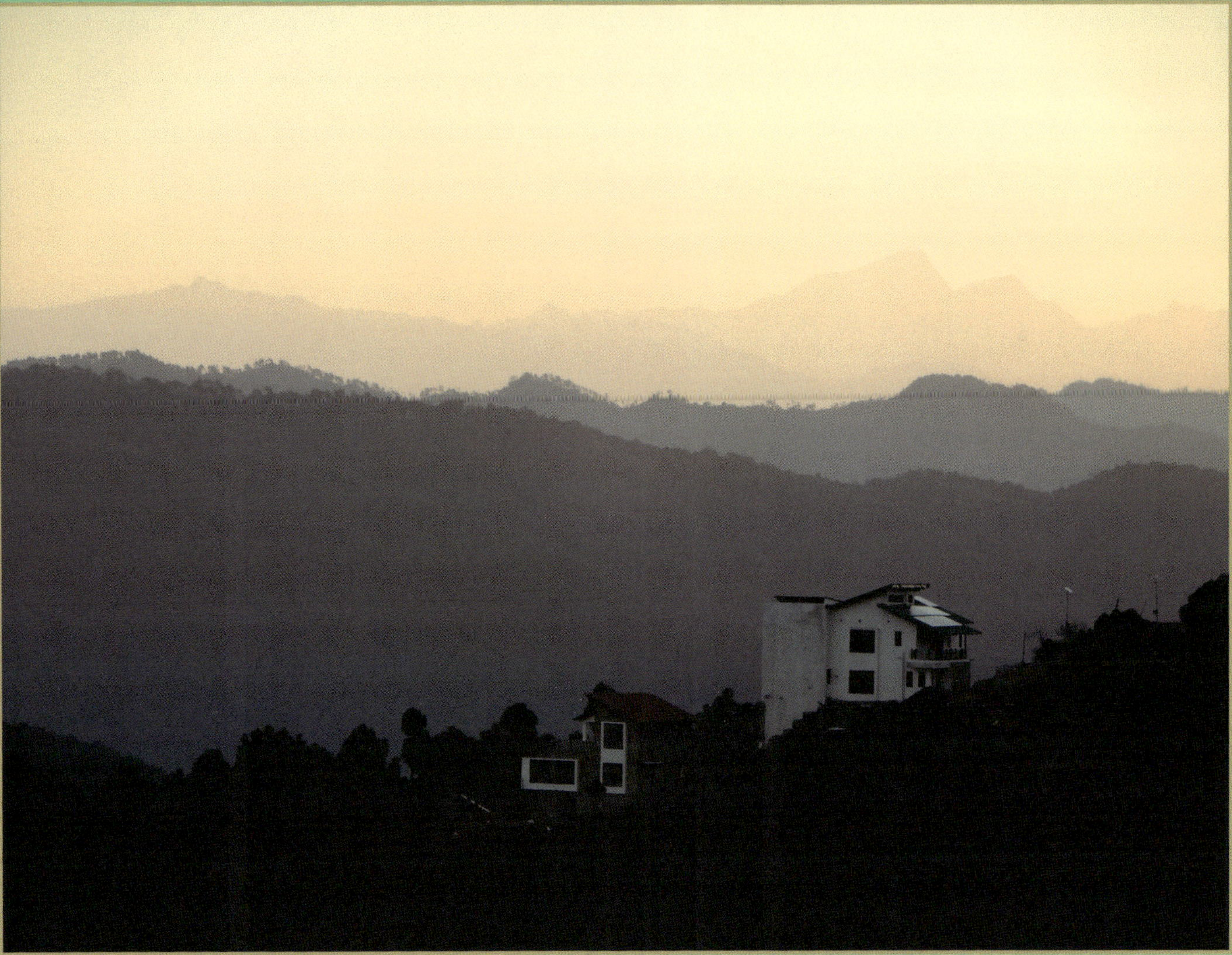

The Wings of My Husband

I understand suddenly my peril
My gossamer wings used to fly alongside my husband's
His path was my path
His direction was my direction

What to do now as I sit in this tree
And my husband's wings are nowhere to be seen?

I shall sit and wait for the wind
Waiting to see him soar above me
And then I shall take flight again.

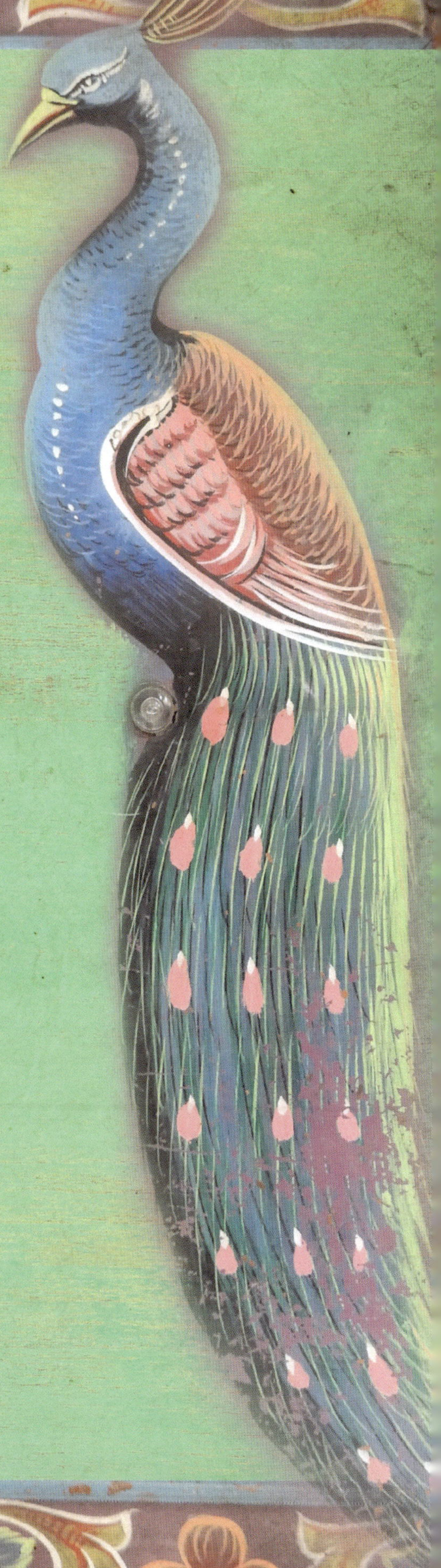

Day 6

(Ranikhet to Nainital)

I wake up at 4 am as usual to make tea in my room and do my usual one to two hours of journal writing. The hotel room is very cold. I am sitting with a lonely heater set on a small round table about 2 feet away. The lonely heater is trying to heat the vast expanse of this cavernous room. But all of that is offset by the incredible Himalaya Mountain view as I open the heavy wooden door to the outside balcony. The early sun has cast an incredible light on the tallest mountains of the distant ridge; the entire ridge is shining with pink white snow. The day before I left on this trip, I was drawn into my cluttered meditation room. I stood wondering why I was here and then my gaze focused on an empty journal book. Of course, it was my husband sending a thought to me "Go and write your journal as usual on this trip." And now I am writing in my journal, taking pictures, writing poetry, and my heart has warmed again. Waiting later in the lobby for Santosh, I pick up a copy of "An Autobiography of a Yogi" and read about the suffusement of light into a student from a master yogi. I determine to buy this book and read it on this trip.

Santosh, Gajendra and myself set off for Nainital, an approximately three-hour drive through mountain village after mountain village. The houses in these villages are again brightly colored in greens and pinks, like flowers sitting brightly on the sides of mountains. I feel like I truly am in the Land of the Gods. The spiritual essence is everywhere. We stop at a viewpoint where I see cascading farm terraces etching every mountainside.

Along the way, we stop at Kainchi Dham temple, a colorful temple by a mountain stream with clear, fresh looking mountain water and surrounding lush hills. An old woman puts her hands in prayer to me and I step to her and place my hands on hers and look deeply into her loving and old eyes. We share a moment of togetherness and sanctity, one heart to another. The temple itself is small with several buildings housing various Gods and Goddesses who are living within their chambers and who are fed and clothed and have beds and couches. A temple is not found within a home; there you will find revered statues but these are not the living entities found within the temple. Before entering, Santosh and I stand on the walkway listening to the prayers and bells. I look at the pure running stream and feel the sunshine warmth on the temple and valley greenery. It is a perfect moment, I think, in time. The land is very sweet.

We carry on to Nainital, a picturesque and quaint city. While in my room at the elegant European-style Naini Retreat hotel, I hear thunder on the roof and look outside. It is a troupe of fun-loving monkeys traipsing across the rooftops of the resort buildings; they look like white macaques but I am certainly no expert. And yes, central heating! I am home!

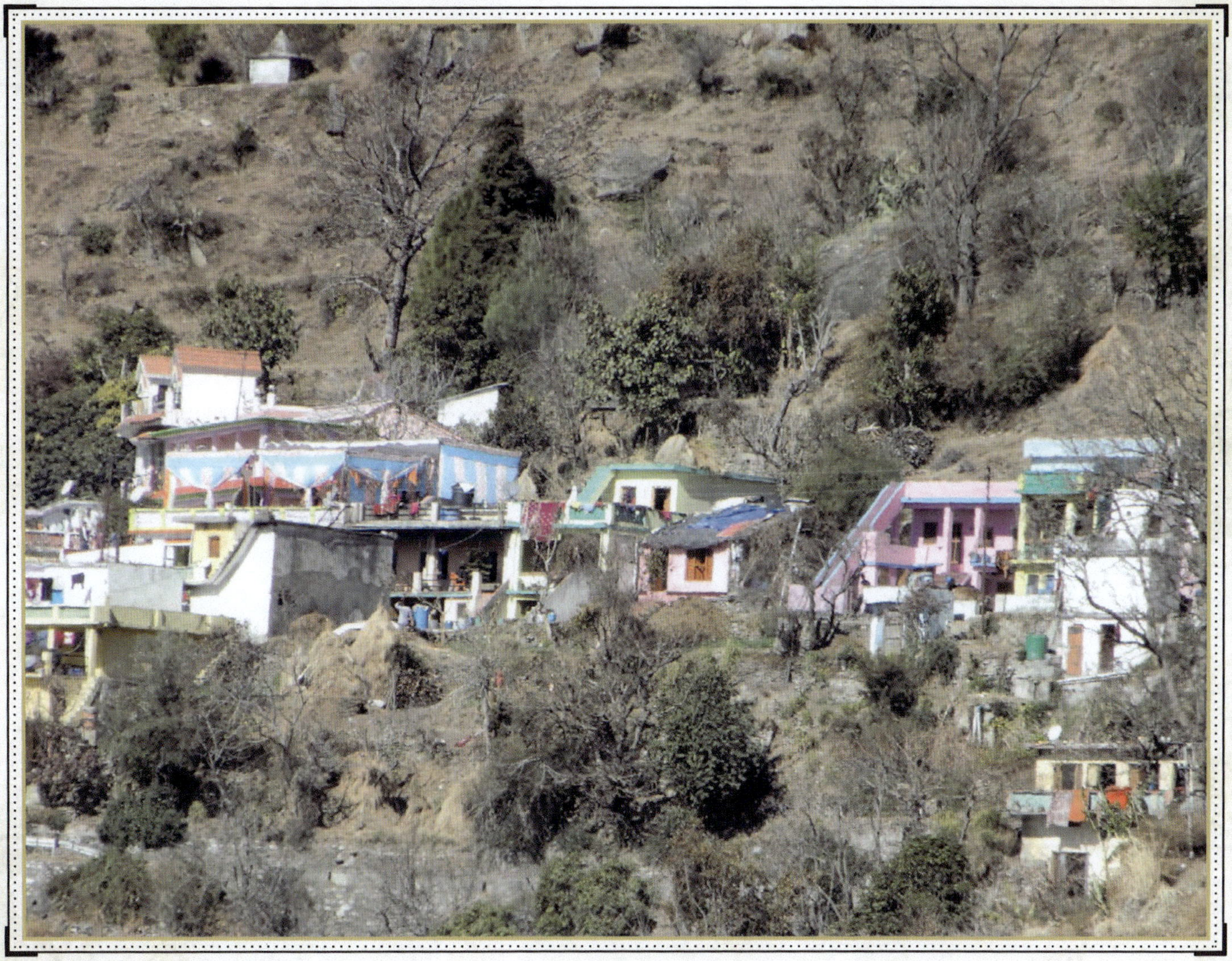

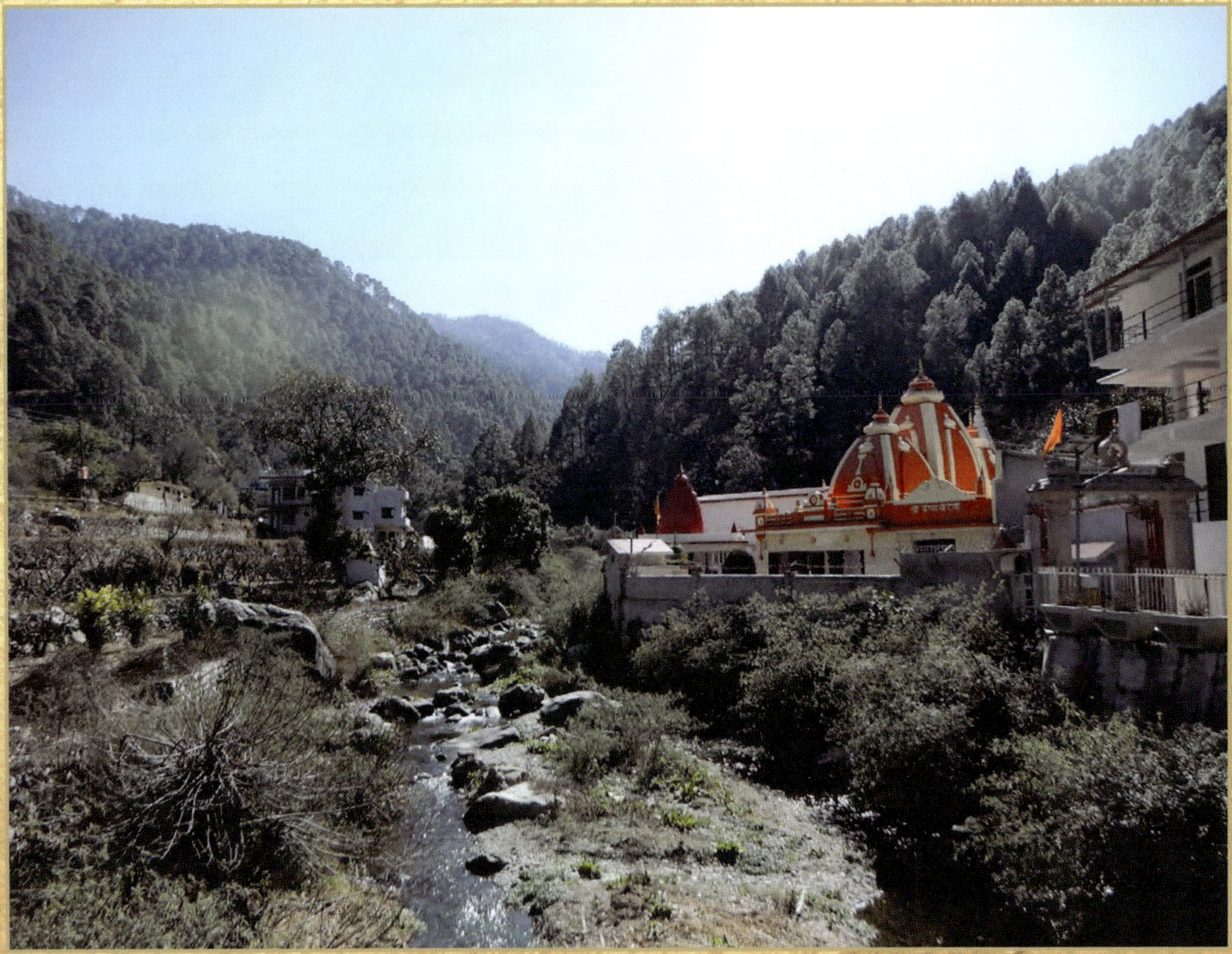

The Fragrance of Love

What is this old age stage?
No husband
Lots of sitting
I see me at the temples
Old women standing quietly
In prayer, in devotion
Women sitting quietly
Their work is done
Now their spirit is the essence
That fills the air
With fragrant love

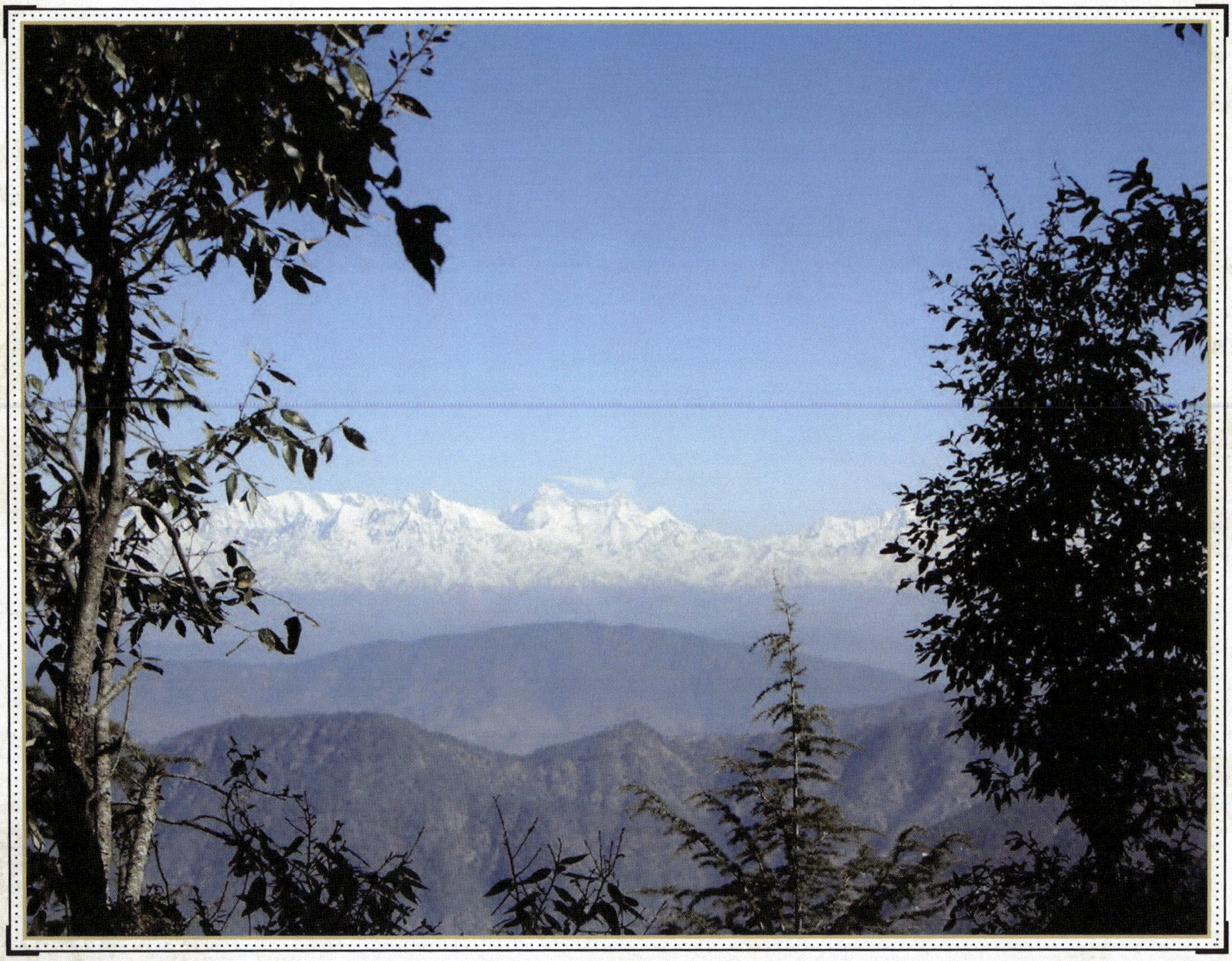

Day 7 and 8

(Nainital)

My habit on this trip is to wake at 4 am, write in my journal and then order breakfast at 8 am. I was thinking the other day about the number 4. It was 4 pm that Kelly and I got married. And we had 40 years together. I like the number 4, and for Kelly, it was the number 7. Sometimes I will get a thought of Kelly and I will look over and the clock will say 7:17 so it is a way of telling me his presence is with me.

Today, Santosh takes me to the Naini Deva temple by Nainital lake. I ring bells and light incense in memory of Kelly. Three Hindu priests are seated in cross-legged position at the lake edge, giving blessings to lake visitors. The lake is considered sacred and created due to the falling of Devi Sati's left eye at this spot. Visitors face the lake and worship with coconut and incense. One priest blesses me with a bindi and motions me to swallow a tablespoon of sacred lake water set in a metal spoon. My logical mind immediately wonders about how safe this will be, but my mystical mind accepts the offering. I have the immediate feeling that even if I get sick, ultimately, I will be stronger for taking this water. We walk along a colorful promenade with lots of shops and we have coffee in a second-floor shop overlooking the lake. I have iced coffee and as I crunch on an ice cube, I remember about not having ice cubes as the water is from general use tap water and not bottled water.

It is a pleasant casual day. Santosh and Gajendra drop me off at the hotel. I head into the courtyard and eat vegies over rice in bright but not too hot sunshine. The moment is perfect and I start to read "Autobiography of a Yogi" as I had picked up the book at a local bookstore after our coffee. Later at night when there is noise in the hallway and with my eyes closed, I see a sudden white explosion of light in my 3rd eye. It is like a transformer has blown and there is no other effect after this. My curtains are closed and I can think of no explanation.

The next day, I am very ill and spend the entire day in bed. Good thing it is not a travelling day. Periodically, I think of how wonderful it was to have my closest companion, my husband, to look after me for 40 years and be by my side for all my ups and downs.

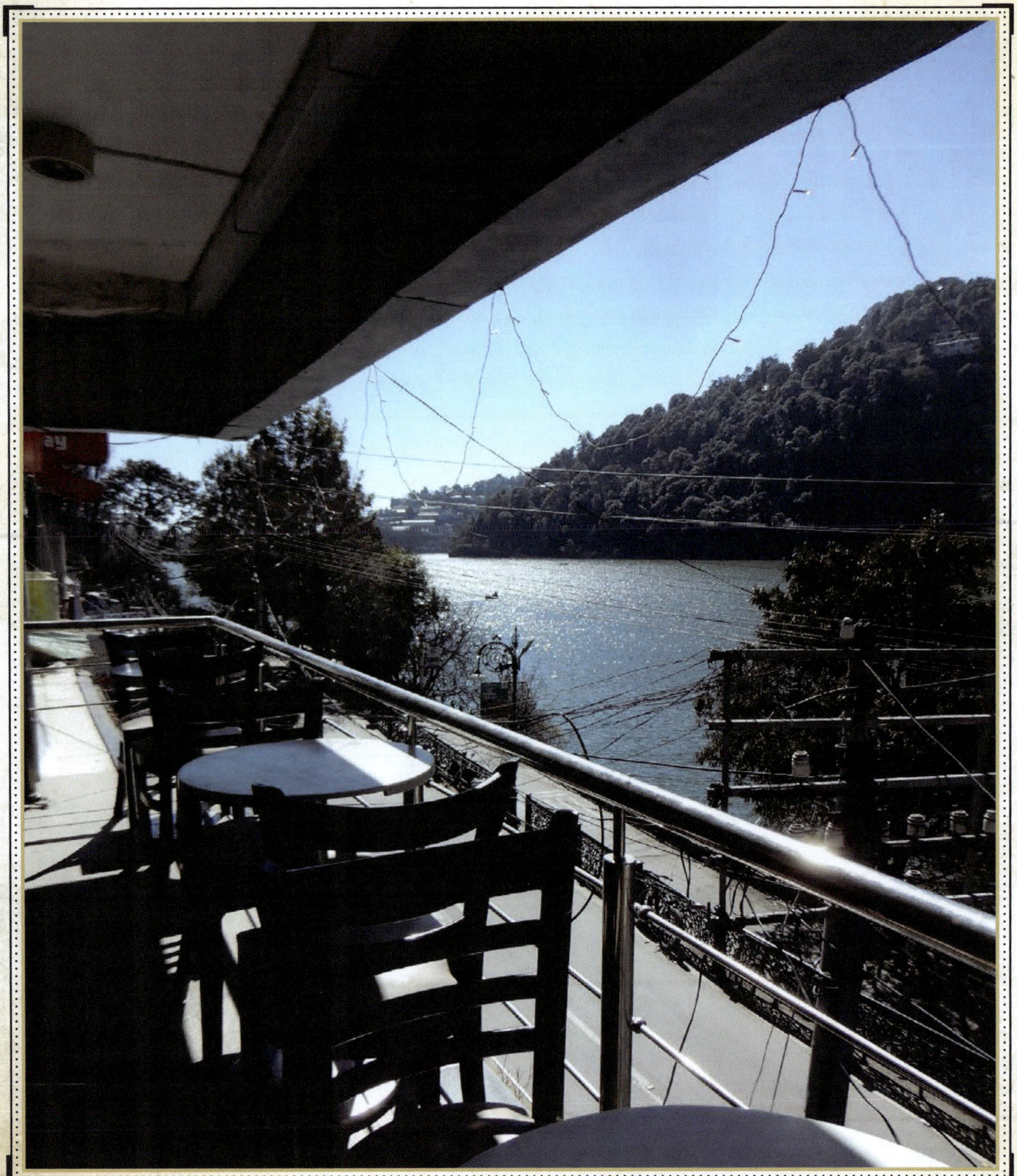

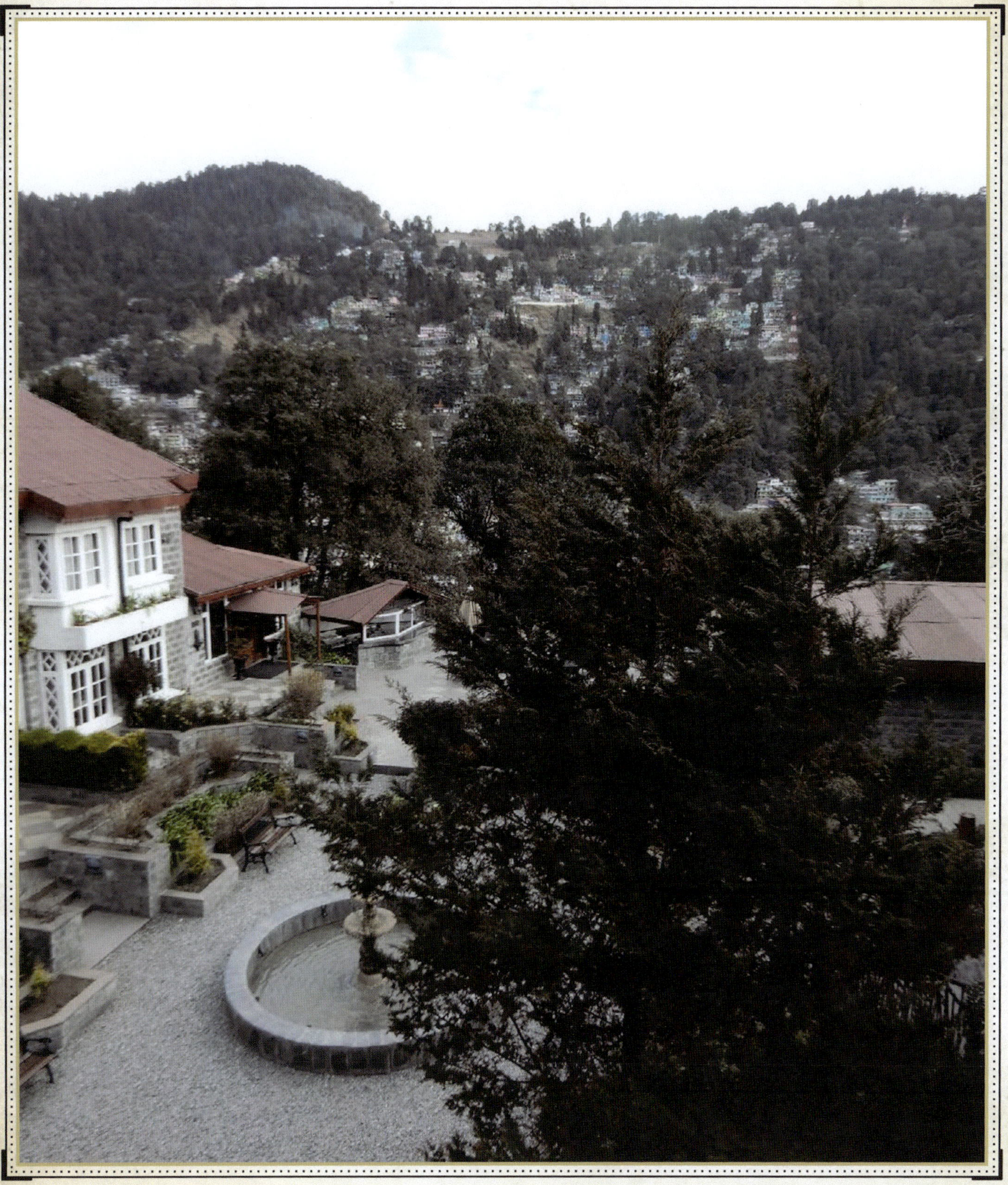

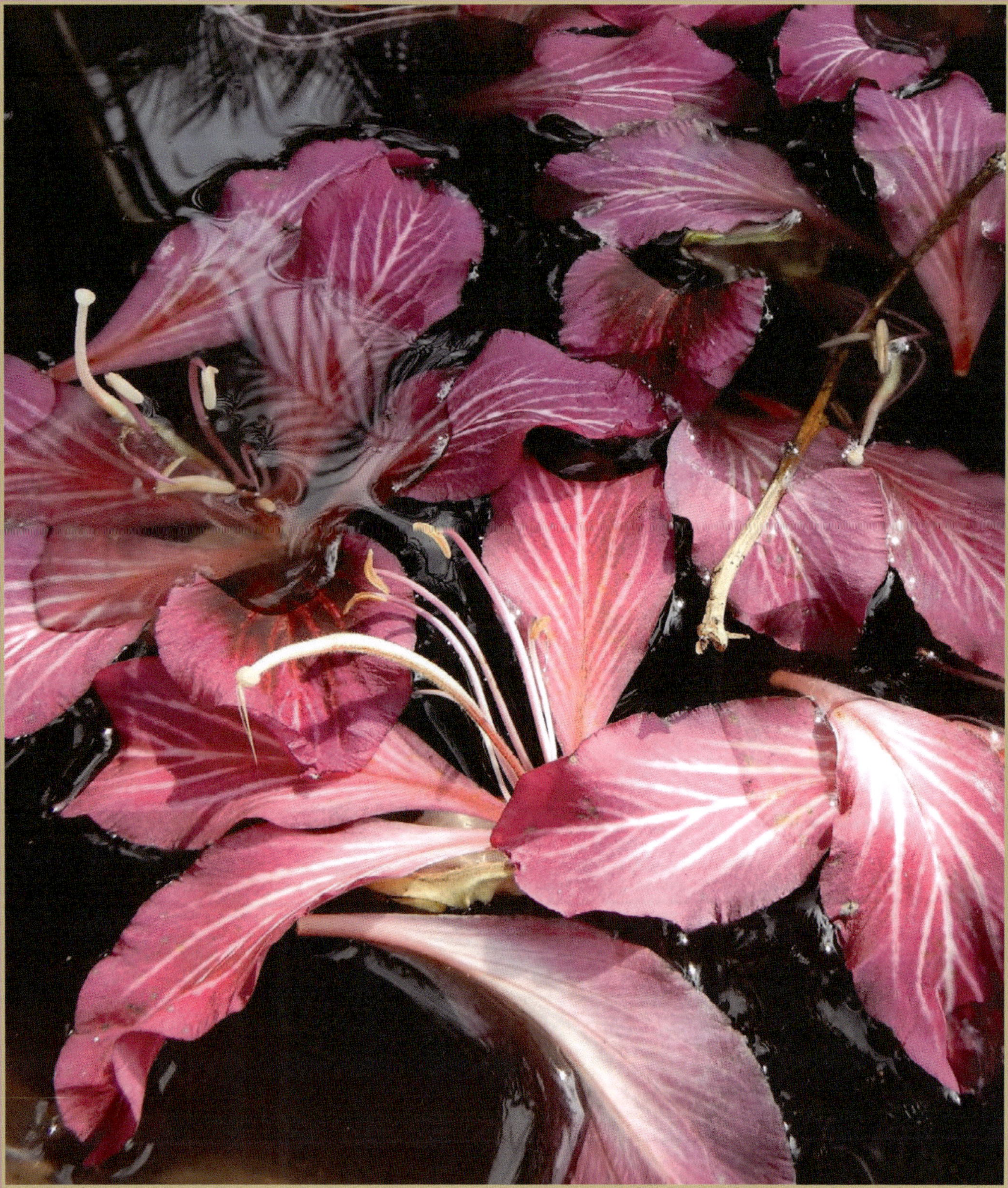

Day 9

(Nainital to Corbett National Park)

The wind is howling outside and creates a clacking noise against the metal roof. This is the weather of mountains and valleys. I hear outside the Hindu priests chanting and ringing bells. An occasional bird chirps. I am feeling better and think it was the ice cubes, and if it was the sacred lake water, I feel I have gained a spiritual strength in my body.

I am starting to descend again into my new life without a partner, and I really do not know my path now. The wind is up, a monkey runs along the aluminum roof above me, and my tears fall.

Santosh, Gajendra and I proceed through another beautiful mountain pass. The hills are starting to bloom. A monkey with a black face and white fur stares in curiosity at us as we pass by. We are on our way to Corbett National Park, one of many parks dedicated to saving the Indian tiger. Before the park, we stop at a village shop and they make a delicious brew of ginger tea. The villagers are harvesting their sugar cane crop and a truck passes us fully loaded with sugar cane stalks stacked at 90 degrees to the flat bed on which they rest and covering more than half the road, they are so long.

My next resort, The Golden Tusk, is brimming with plants and trees and birds. I sit at an outside table and continue with "Autobiography of a Yogi".

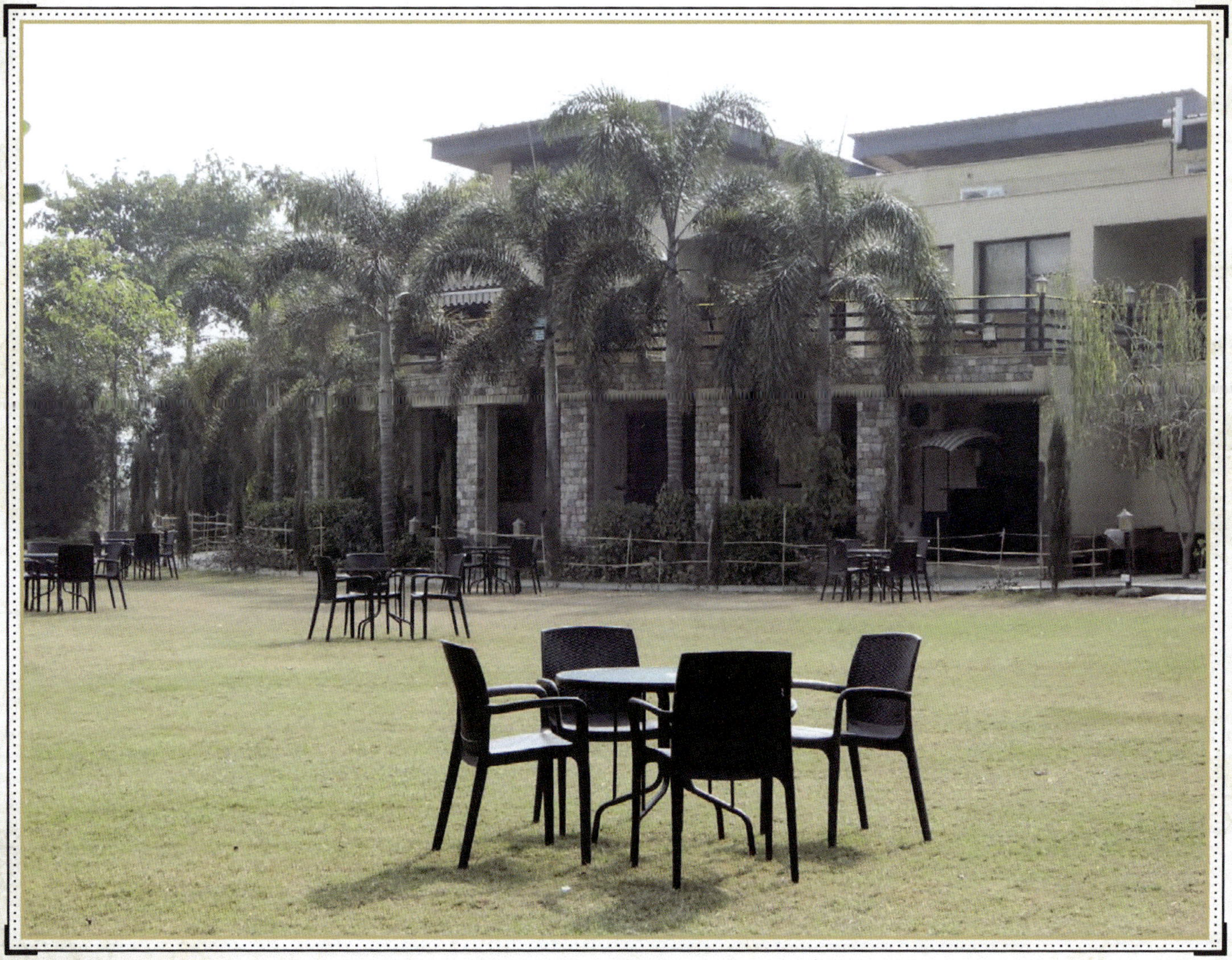

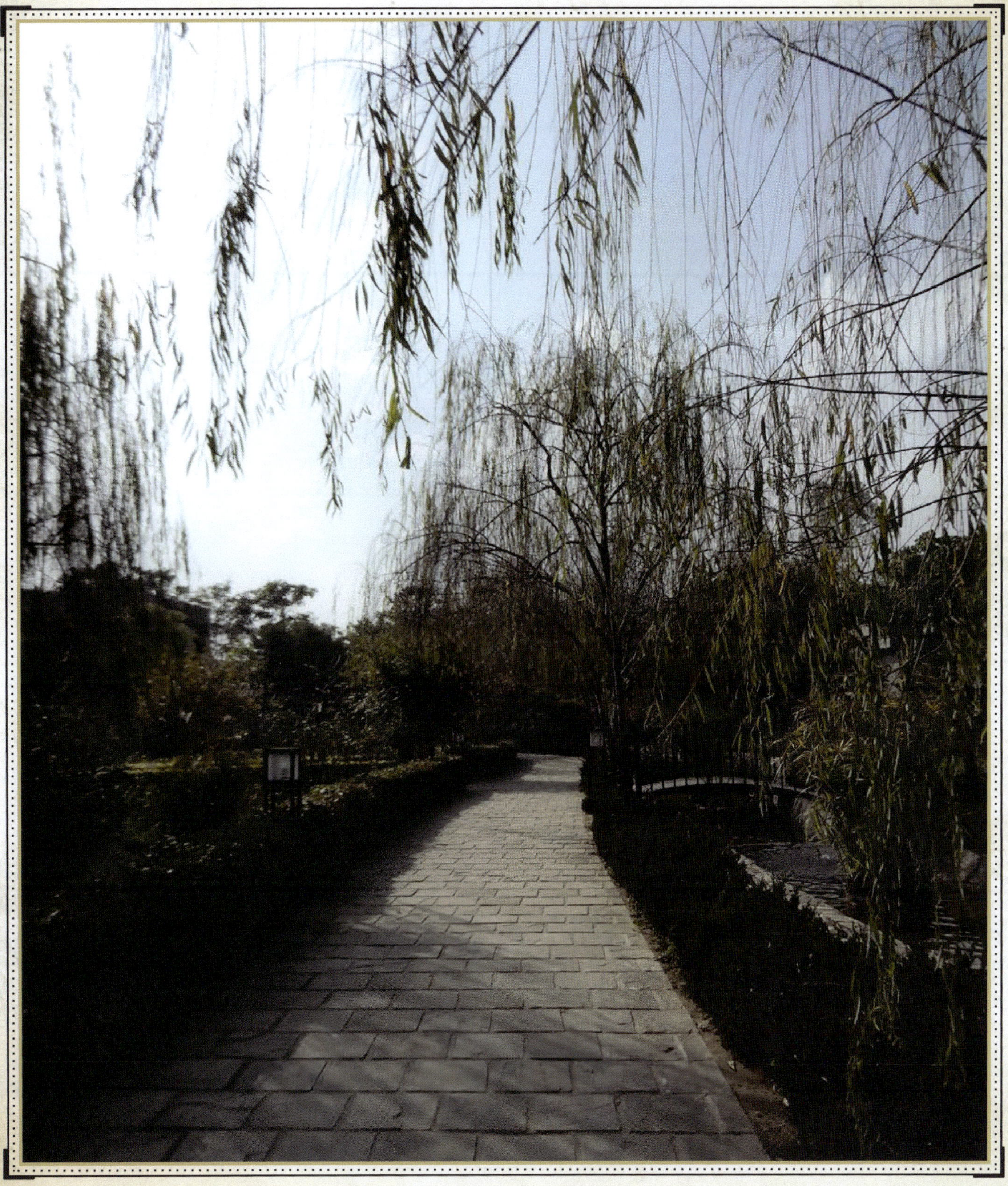

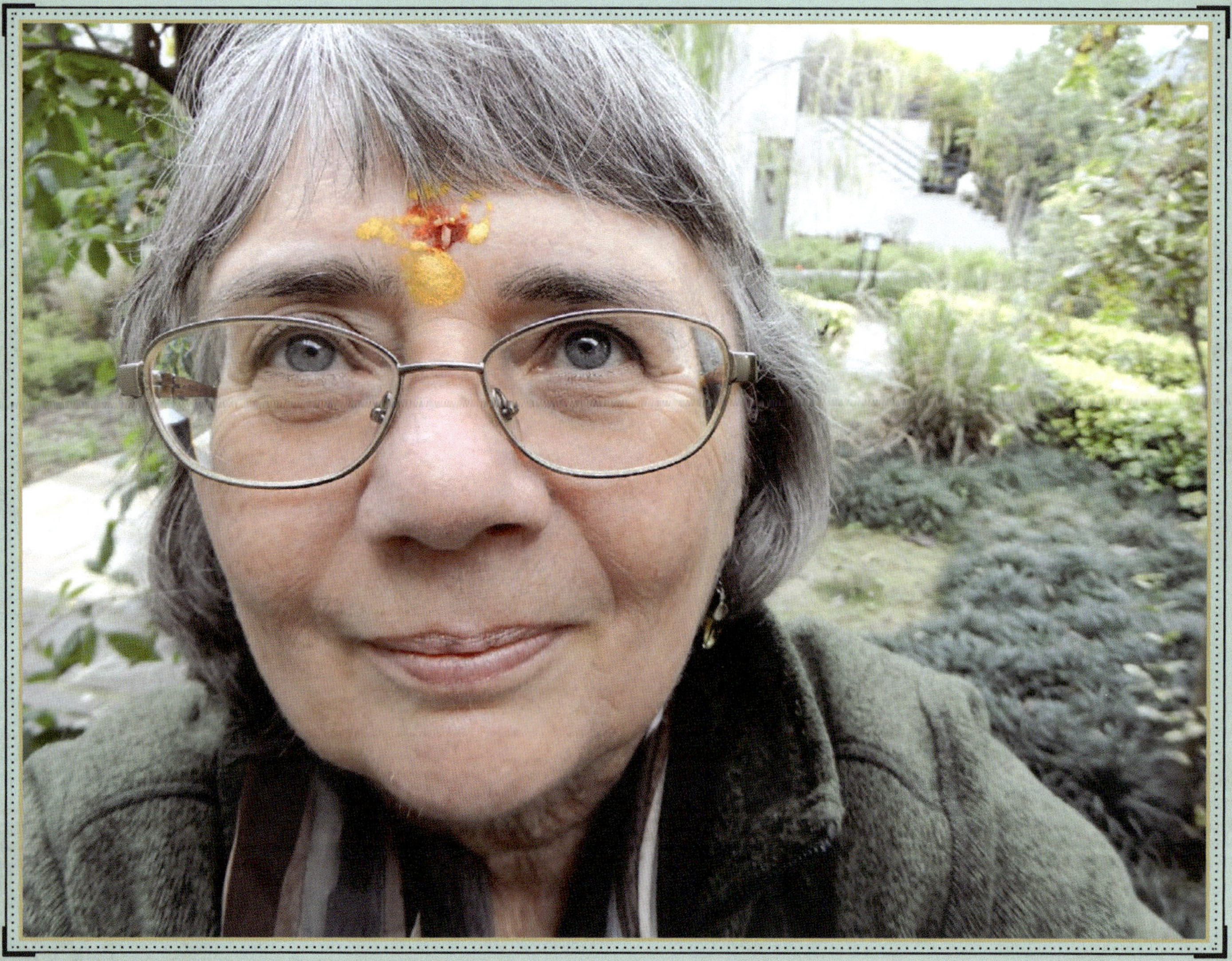

Today, I Have Invited Shiva To Tea

Today, I sent out my thought
High into the mountains
Where the wild man lives

Today, I have invited Shiva to tea
I am hoping he takes time from
His boundless energies
To sit with me and listen
As I express my soul to him

His form is pure energy
I am hoping he does not break my delicate vessel
As I pass it to him

Today, I have invited Shiva to tea
Even Gods can be inspired
By the love of a simple woman

Lightning may strike
A vortex of wind may flatten the trees

But just for a moment
It will only be Shiva and me
Touching our cups together
On a high mountain ledge

Day 10

(Corbett National Park)

It is so beautiful here. I wake up to the birds singing and a light mist over the lush green fields. Today, we travel to an ancient temple beside the Kosi River. This is the Garjiya Devi Temple which is a sacred Shakti shrine where Garjiya Devi is the presiding deity. The temple is set on top of a high rock with a vertical drop on one side and with a graduated slope of about 45 degrees on the other. We buy offerings for the Goddess including clothing – a bright red taffeta piece of cloth. We walk up the narrow steep stairway of the graduated slope, to the top. It is a very pure environment mixed with the chanting of devotees, the ringing of bells and the giving of blessings from the priest. On seeing my face, the priest brings out a book telling the story of his father who went to the United States. It is a nice moment of sharing. Santosh and I leave the small temple space and walk around outside looking at the view and then descend back down the narrow staircase. Many singing and laughing school children are now ascending to the top.

Another small temple is close by and it is in a cave so I go through a narrow stone alcove to reach the priest. I wonder who had meditated here many years ago. Once out and having prasad sweets in my pocket, a friendly cow nudges me to be generous. I am a little unsure of what to do and place most of the prasad over to the left on the ground and I walk away while she is eating. I sprinkle my remaining prasad into the moderately flowing clear river and make a wish for the happiness of the world. A single marigold floats by past me. Santosh and I head further downstream where there are many more people sitting on rocks. As I choose a rock to sit on, Santosh gets chai. Gajendra also joins us briefly. Beside us a family group of about ten, including an older grandmother and grandfather, mother, priest and sisters, are in a circle giving blessings to a young man who is about to get married in the next few days. It is a special event and includes each family member going down to the river to put their hands in the water to bathe and receive blessings from the water. They bring back water to the young man from their hands to his, also as a blessing.

There are water birds and one brown cow that roams through and it is all just a part of the energy of the moment. What a special place. I feel completely at peace and happy. While on the rock, briefly on my own, I close my eyes and do a meditation in my mind's eye, where the world is moving all around me, but I am completely still in the centre. Later that day, after I return and am settled in my room, I hear thunder, and rain begins. Somehow, I feel I have started a second phase of my journey into the mountains to visit Shiva.

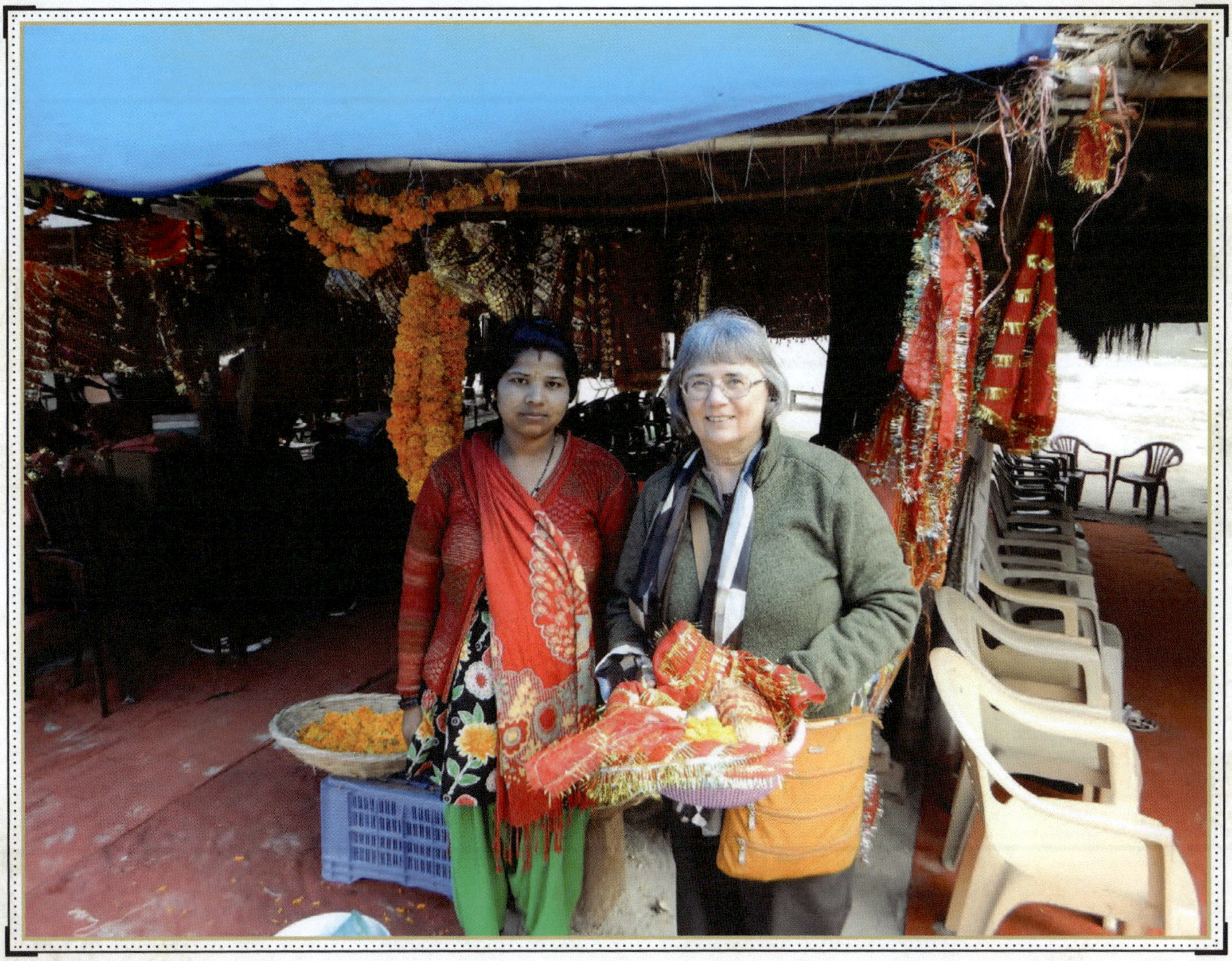

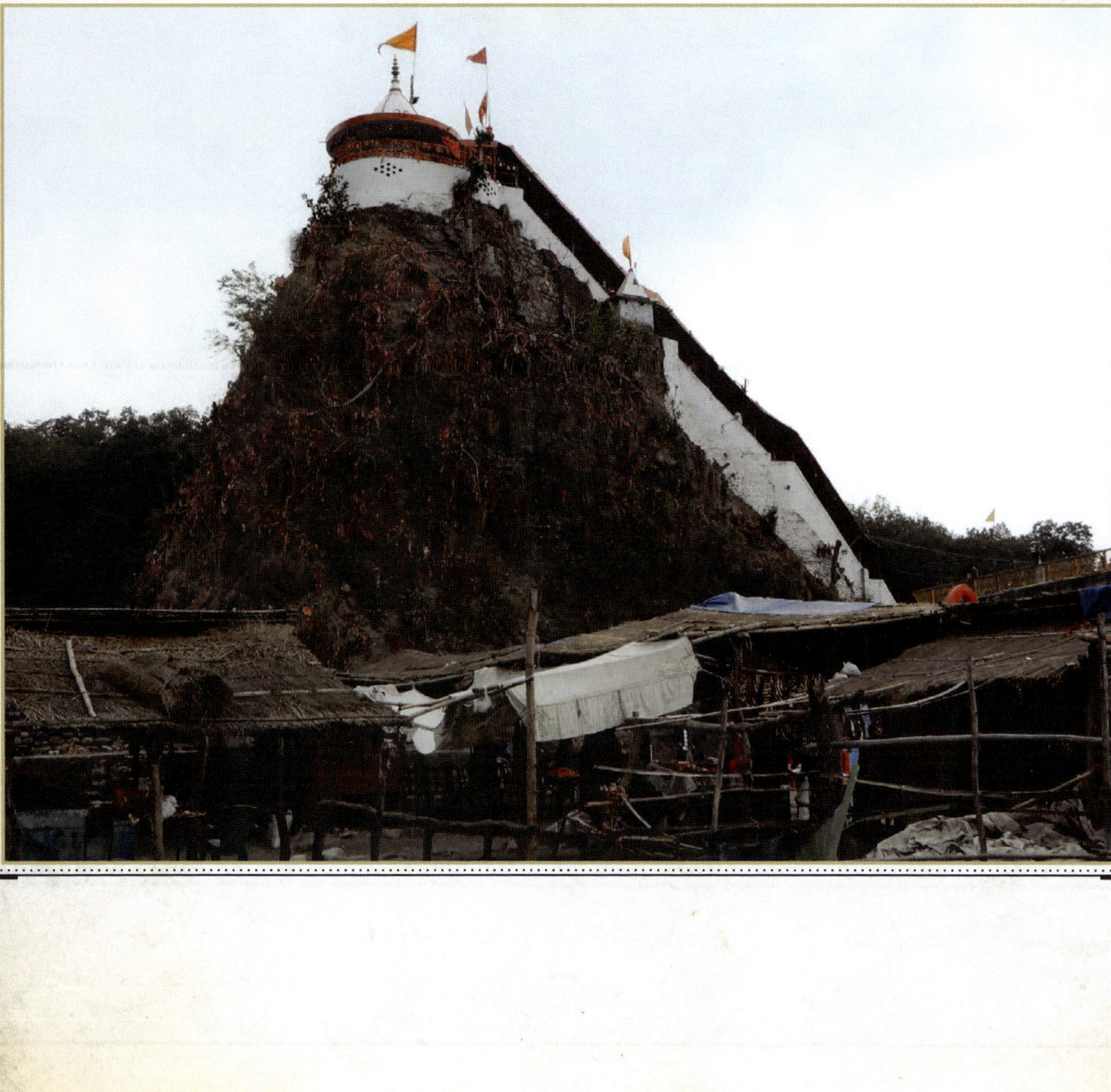

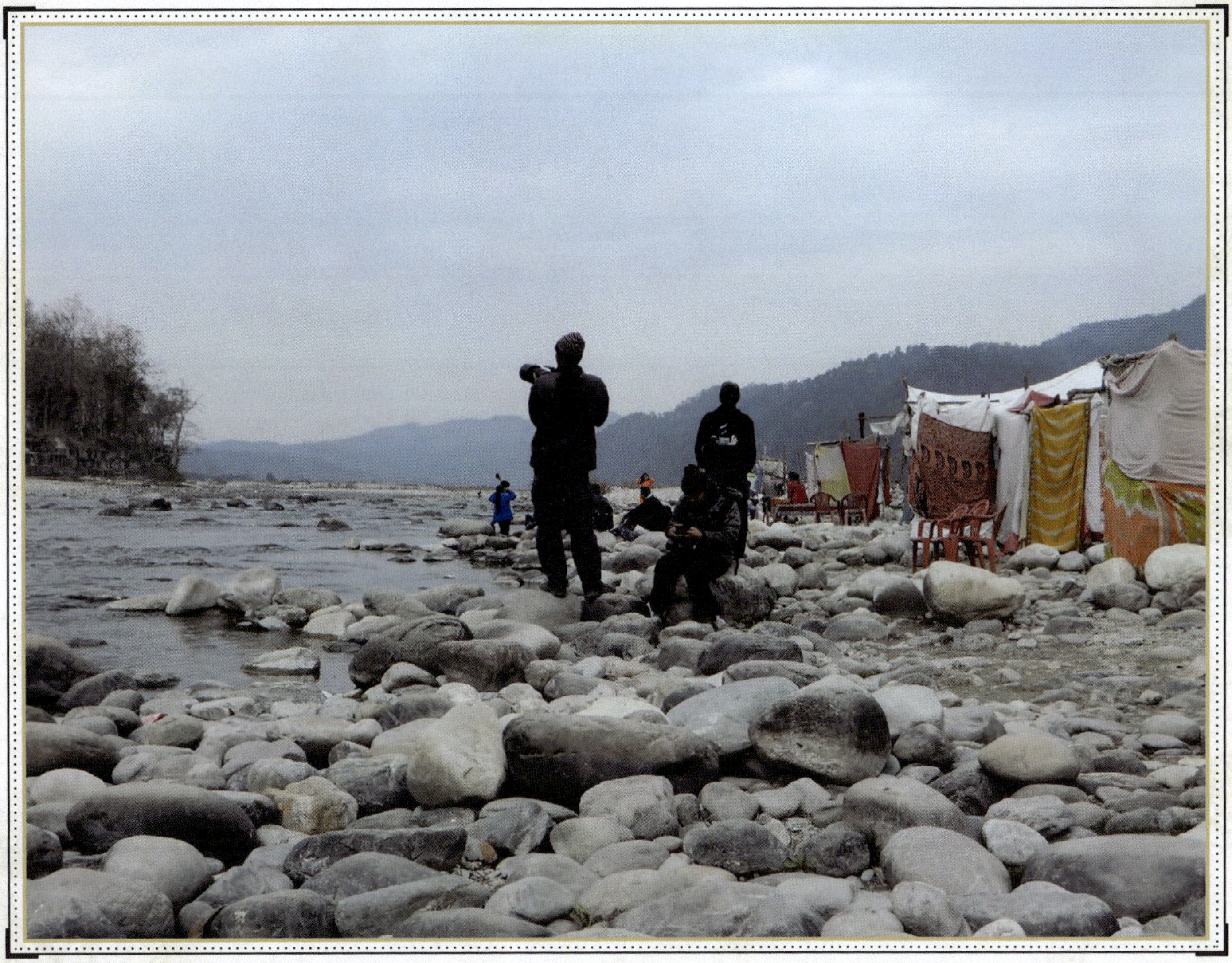

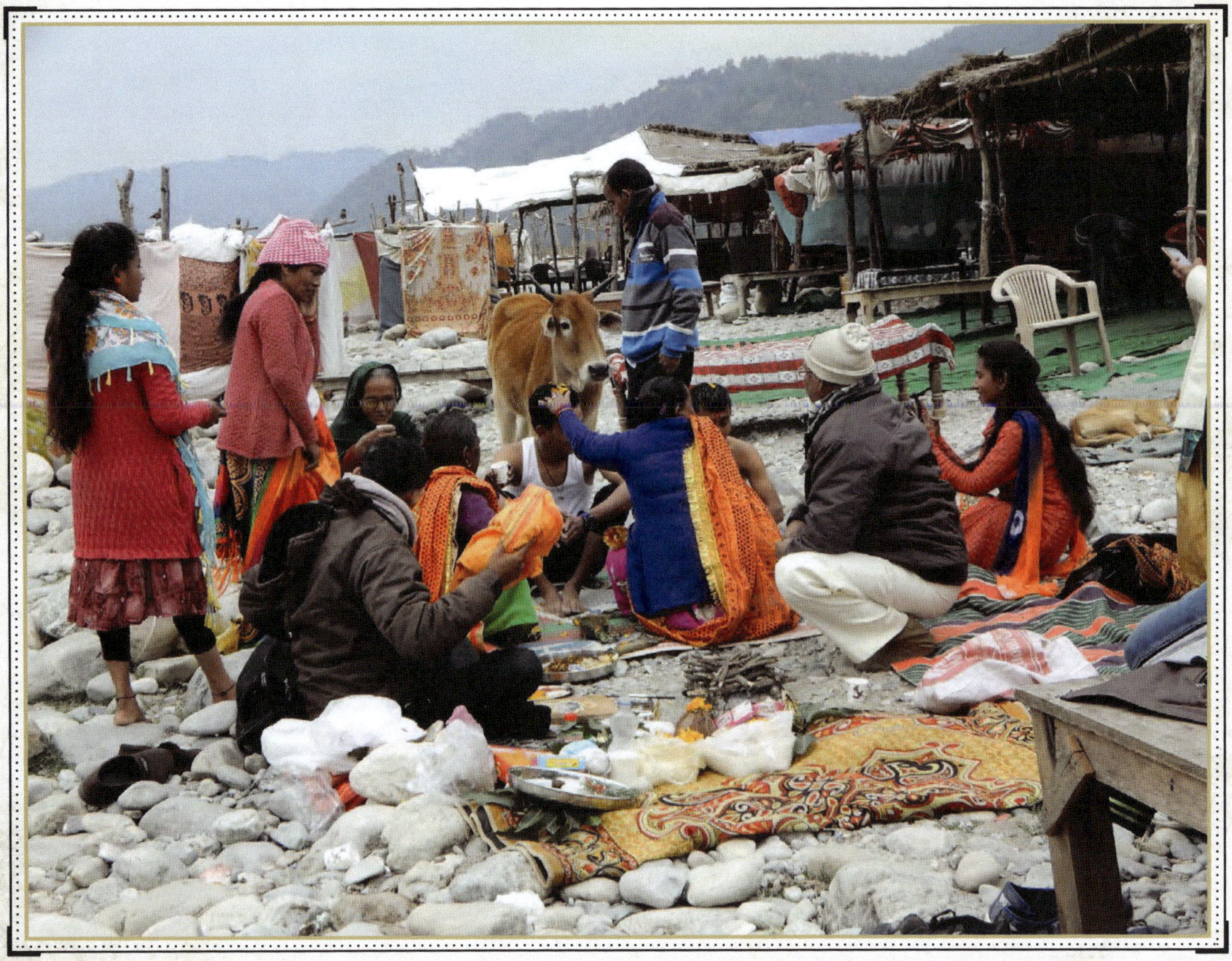

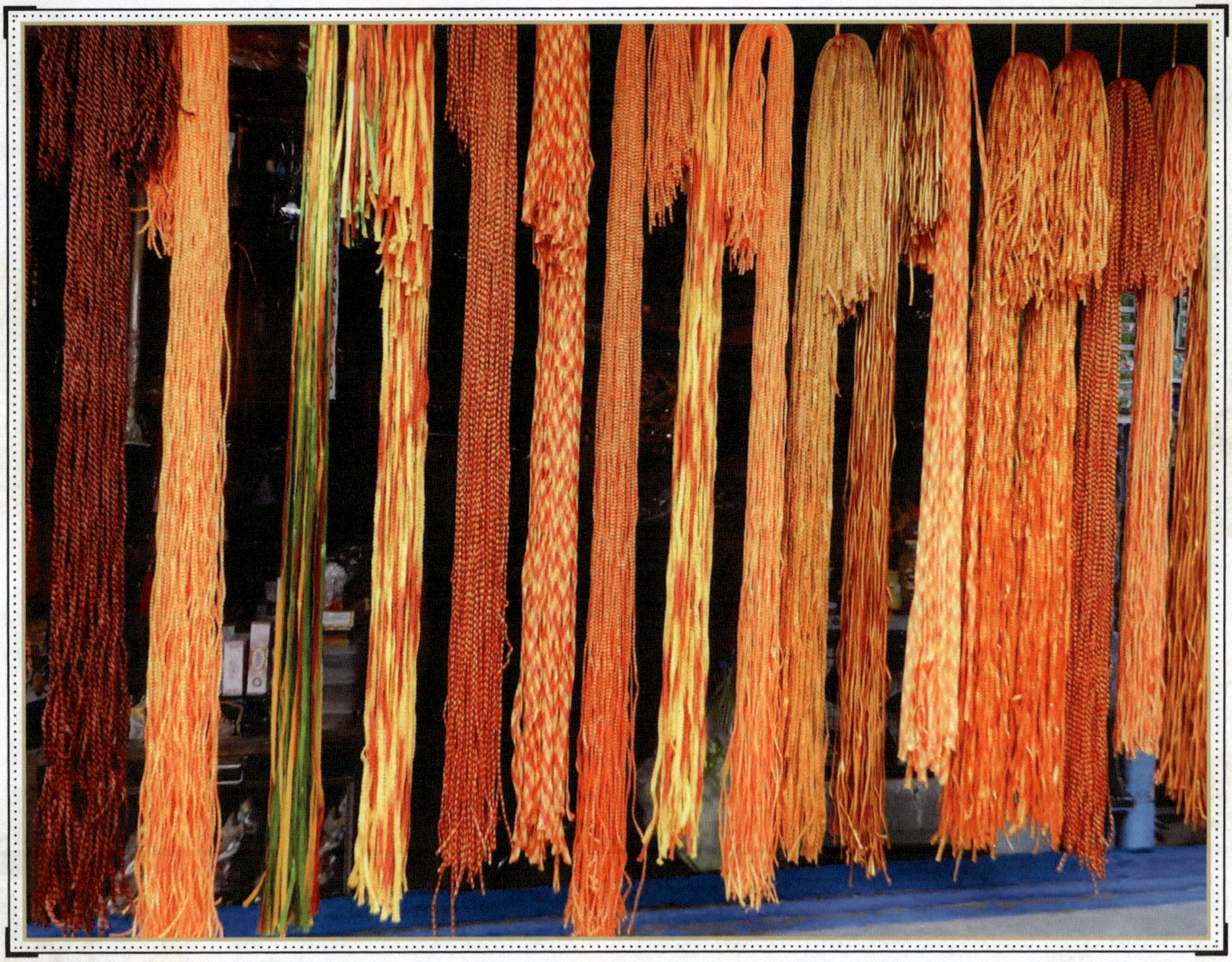

Dhaba Time

Sudden stop
Next to clean dhaba
Horns continuous beside us

A steaming na'an is brought out
Chai for me
Calmness in busyness

An idle line of poetry
To pass the time.
I am grateful for
My concentrated thought
To forget the noise around me
Briefly

Day 11

(Corbett to Lansdowne)

I have had an odd and disturbing dream of Kelly. He has the symptoms of a heart attack. I call 911 but the operator is slow and, in the meantime, Kelly gets up and starts walking up a hill against my protestations. I am so scared for him but he is out of control. He joins another man and drinks liquid out of what looks like an alcohol still. He shows me that there is actually no alcohol in the mix. His wild and free nature has me so upset in the dream, but as I sit here writing the journal, I think it is my own absorption of the stories of Shiva, and reading of Paramahansa Yogananda, author of "Autobiography of a Yogi", who is himself going to the mountains to meet a master.

It is morning and the rolling thunder and monsoon-like rains continue. I wonder how safe the mountain roads will be for rock slides and lightning on our six-hour journey. We begin our journey and throughout it, the roads are safe and the sun soon shines. Gajendra has placed ten marigolds on the front dash. They are so colorful and I am sure their energy is adding to the good luck of the trip. We pass many sugar cane trucks taking their harvest to the mill. The houses are brightly colored in blues, lavender and orange. There has been heavy snowfall in the areas of Kausani that we had just travelled through in previous days. And heavy rain will close the schools for two days. On the busy but narrow roads to the foothills of Lansdowne, there are horse-pulled carriages hauling heavy items of flour and rice just like they must have done hundreds of years ago. We carry on to a very interesting bazaar area at the foothills of our climb. The markets are teeming with people and colourful quilts and shawls. The streets seem like pandemonium but everyone moves around each other easily. Then the climb begins and immediately, a sweetness enters the air. The forest reappears as dense Himalayan pines mixed with newly blooming bushes. I see a holy man dressed only in black rather than the usual saffron robes. Santosh tells me he is most likely a devotee of another form of Shiva. The hill climbs continuously and we are soon high up into the mountains with the beautiful river Kho beside us adding lushness. My new hotel, Kasang Regency Hill Resort, is on the edge of the side of a mountain. Its balcony has a stunning view of the Himalayas.

I prepare my three quilts, two hats, two pairs of socks and gloves, and head to bed early. I awake to a rumble of thunder in the distance at about 9 pm. The rumble is continuous and soon is joined by sheets of lightning. We are so high up that we are in the lightning production zone. As the storm goes on for hours and hours, I realize I am in a super cell of electrical voltage. I think the hotel takes a direct hit. I am mentally calculating if the roof will blow off, the winds are that extreme. The storm disintegrates to monsoon rain and I am finally able to rest.

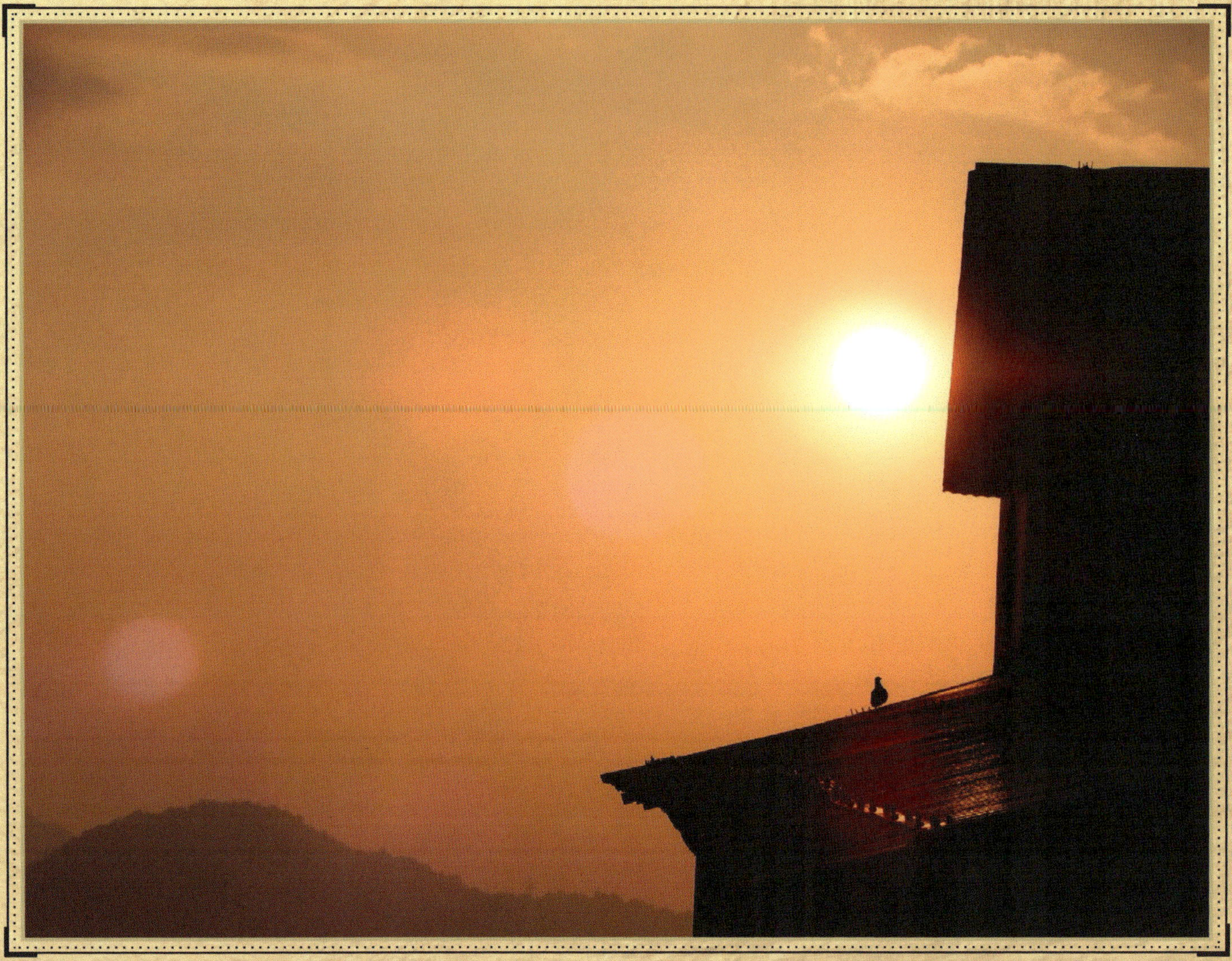

A Request to You, Dear Shiva

Dear Shiva, I have a request for you
I had asked you to tea a few days ago
I forgot to mention
Please come in your humble form

Last night, you came in full form
Your power erupted in blazes of light
So bright, I thought my life would end
You barely spoke and the roof thundered
You barely shook your hair and water
Filled the universe around me.
I huddled under the quilts, dear,
I did not have time to prepare your tea

So next time, dear
Although it was so good to see you
I request your humble form
Like Hanuman on his knees to Mother Sita

Then you can gently place a rose crystal within my mind
And I can sit in meditation state
Wearing a warm green Kausani shawl
While I generate divinity beside your darker mass
And the owls by the stream can share in our adventure

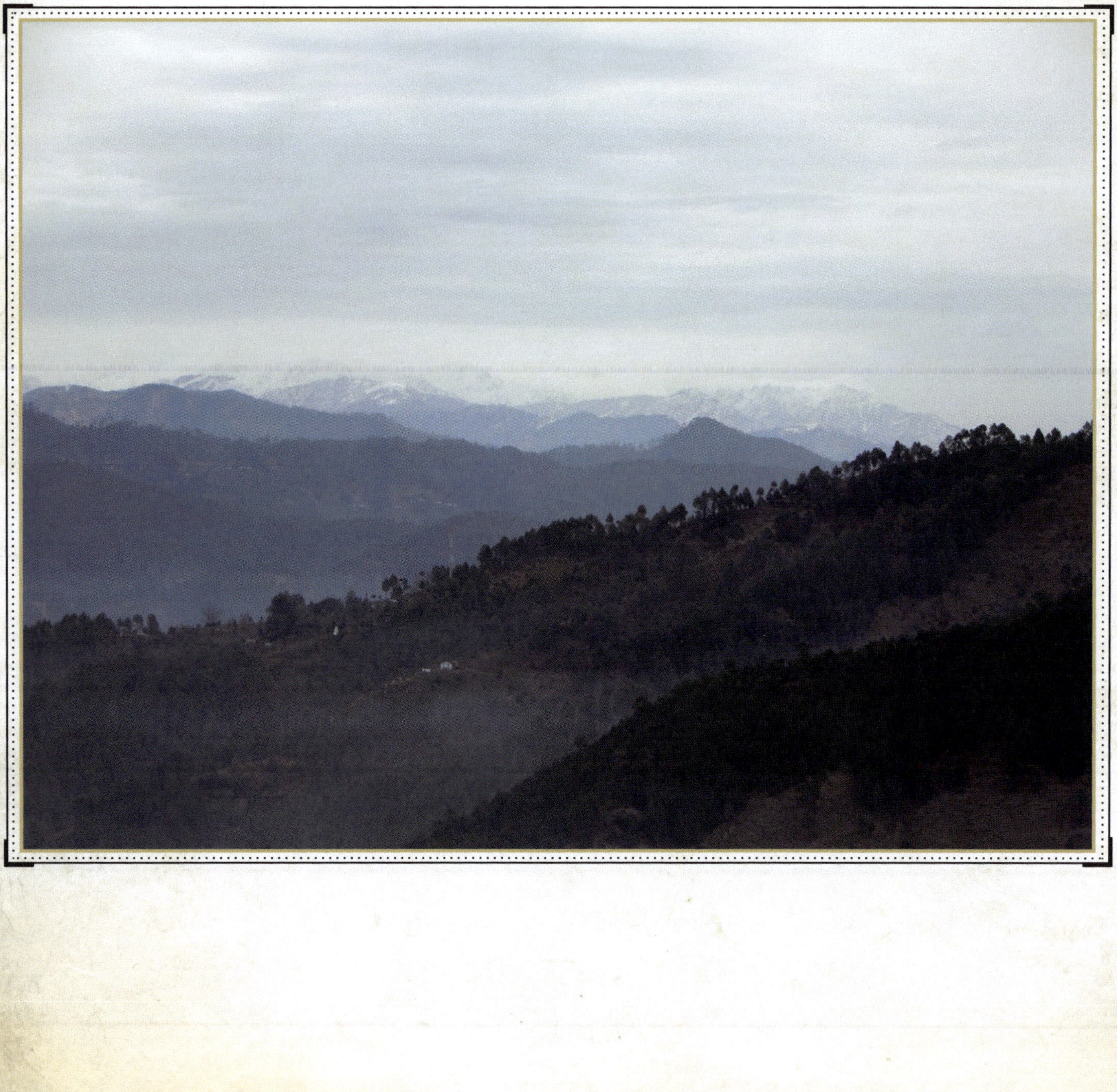

Day 12
(Lansdowne)

At sunrise, I step out onto the balcony. The sun is coming up spreading its warmth and comfort, a welcome relief from the numbing focus on the lightning, thunder, wind and rain of the previous night. The birds are singing; I hear the locals singing and chanting nearby and it is hard to believe the fast metamorphosis of mood.

Today, we strike out to Takeshwar temple devoted to Lord Shiva. Again, it is a long but beautiful journey through the high mountain roads, past singular houses and their farms set upon the steep mountain hillside with the ever-present terraces and cows. Occasional groups of families are doing roadwork on these out-of-the-way mountain roads. Nonetheless, there is a regular public transit system. Again, the day is lovely for this two-hour trip to reach the remote temple. Once we arrive, it is a long walk down a well-established rock trail in mature forest. This area feels ancient and has an old history although the temple is relatively new. We doff our shoes and walk the wet path to the temple. I strike bells on a line to the temple. Inside the actual small space, the priest puts yellow bindis on and gives us prasad. Afterwards, we walk around and are the only visitors to this quiet sacred spot in the woods.

On returning to the hotel, we stop at a clean eatery and order alu paratha - onion, potato and cauliflower stuffed breads. Once I return to my room, I sit restfully on my balcony outside, gazing at the spacious and beautiful Himalayan mountains.

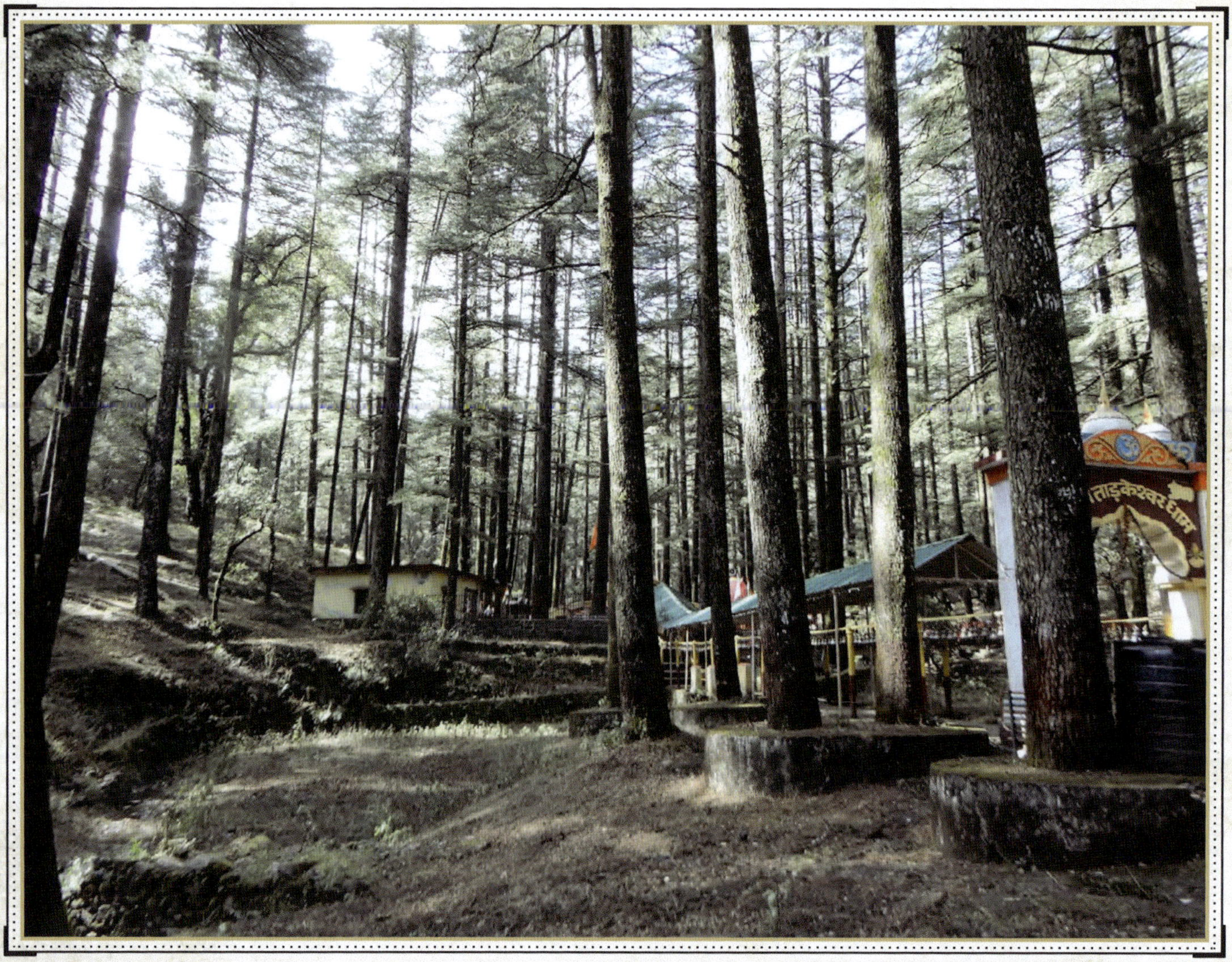

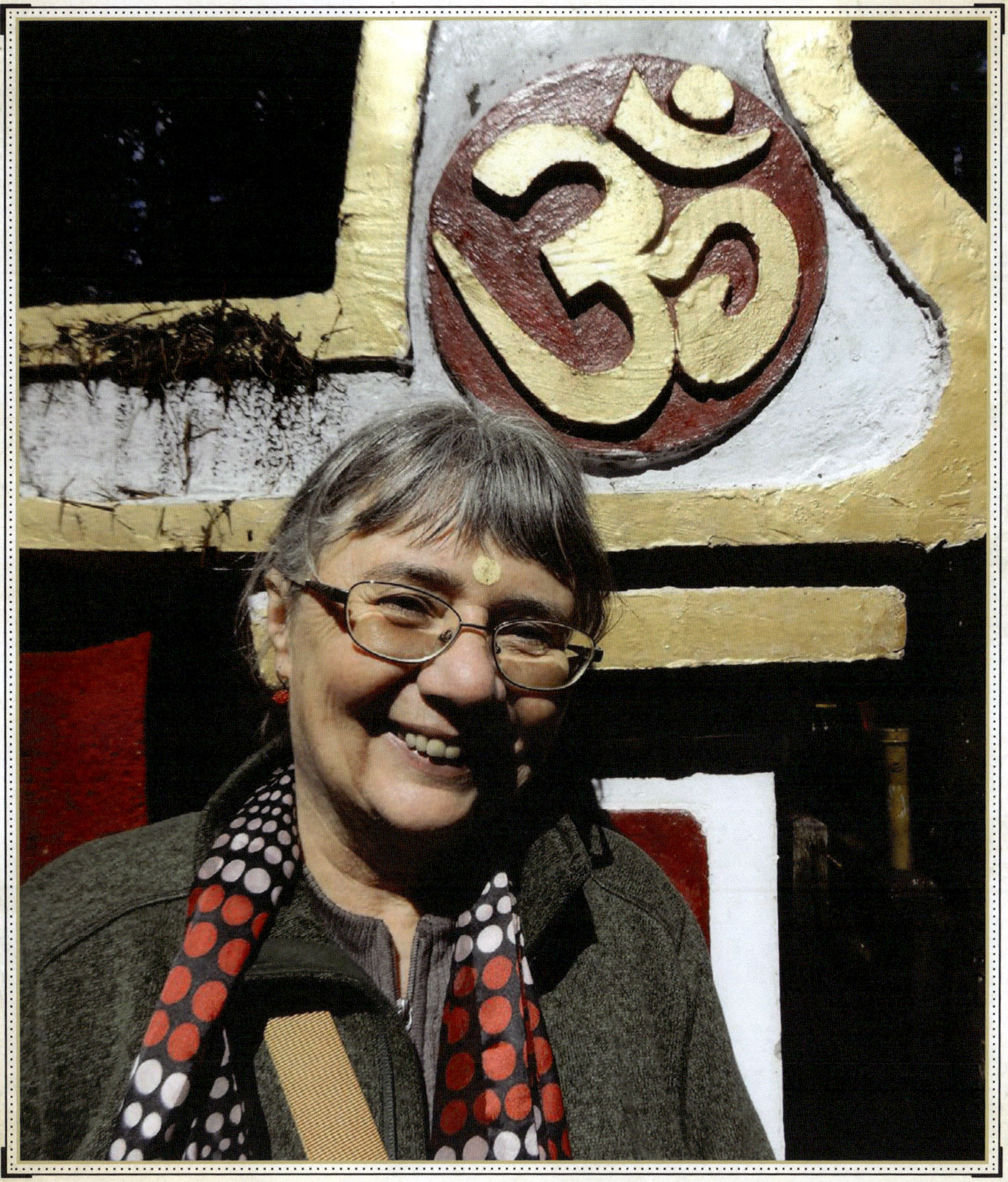

The Signs Are Good

The signs are good, my friend,
Good omens are all around
To take the gateway to God.

Upon chanting Om Namah Shivaya
Many times upon my prayer beads,
A garuda circled towards me
From a distant Himalayan hill top.

Circled through the fog and into
The clear blue sky above me.

Tonight, the sun sank in glorious orange colour
Its radiant orange filling the sky like embers of a fire
About to be lit again.

One hand touches the other in prayer.

The transmission will be pure as we walk the steps
Up to the heavens.

Om Namah Shivaya

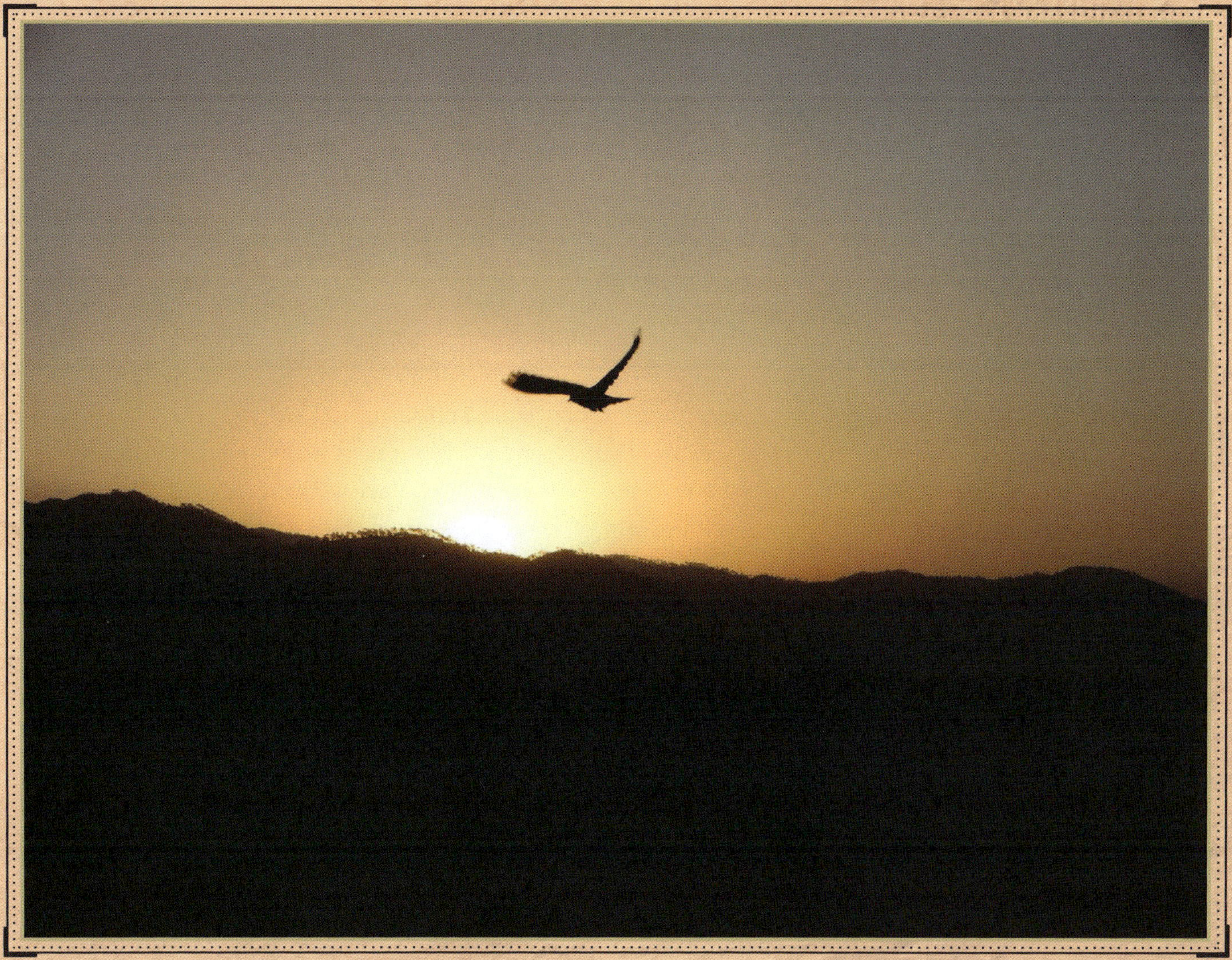

Day 13

(Lansdowne)

I arise early at 5 am and prepare myself for the day. On the balcony, I sit for two hours in a quiet meditative state with my warm, green Kausani shawl around my shoulders. The colours are pink and grey upon the horizon of rolling mountains before the sun comes up. Birds swoop together in the light breeze that shakes the needles of the trees and pushes early clouds through the valleys. The sun gently rises behind the large mountains to the left, music starts in the village and the pigeons start to coo on the roof above me. I have brought two cups of coffee outside so that I can share this moment with Kelly, just as we had shared so many other early morning moments together. I confess I do not know if he is actually here or if he has continued to evolve into a new cycle and I am just the remnants of an age gone by and now no more. I also confess that if he is here, perhaps he is encouraging me to "let go". I have always been able to see clearly into the future for all my life, but now I have no vision, just a great confusion as to my life direction. Shall I shut a door behind me? But in doing so am I committing a grave error of turning my back on the one that I love should he still be there with me in this world and waiting for me on the other side?

Santosh and Gajendra pick me up at 10 am as usual. Today we are heading for Lansdowne to see various tourist stops. First, it is a drive through the army cantonment area and then into the town area of Lansdowne. We stop at Bhula Taal, a quiet lake area which is really water behind an old stone dam. Everything is quiet and peaceful as we are surrounded by nature. There are young couples near us also sitting and enjoying the warm sun. We drive to two churches from the British era in the mid 1800's. It is nice to share some of my childhood church history and knowledge with Santosh, and tell him about the history of the Catholic and Protestant churches, and some shared spirituality that links all peoples – the universal spark of divinity and light within all of us.

Next, we take in Tippin Top, a strategic mountain top area for taking pictures of some of the tallest majestic Himalayan mountains. Finally, we head to where Santosh is staying at a homestay. We enjoy a delicious lunch of potato paratha and a Kurjwali-style vegetable dish with spicy sauce, yogurt and finally chai.

It has been a lovely, relaxing day. In the evening, the sunset is stunningly beautiful with oranges and roses, and it feels like a good omen to be travelling to Haridwar tomorrow, Gateway to God.

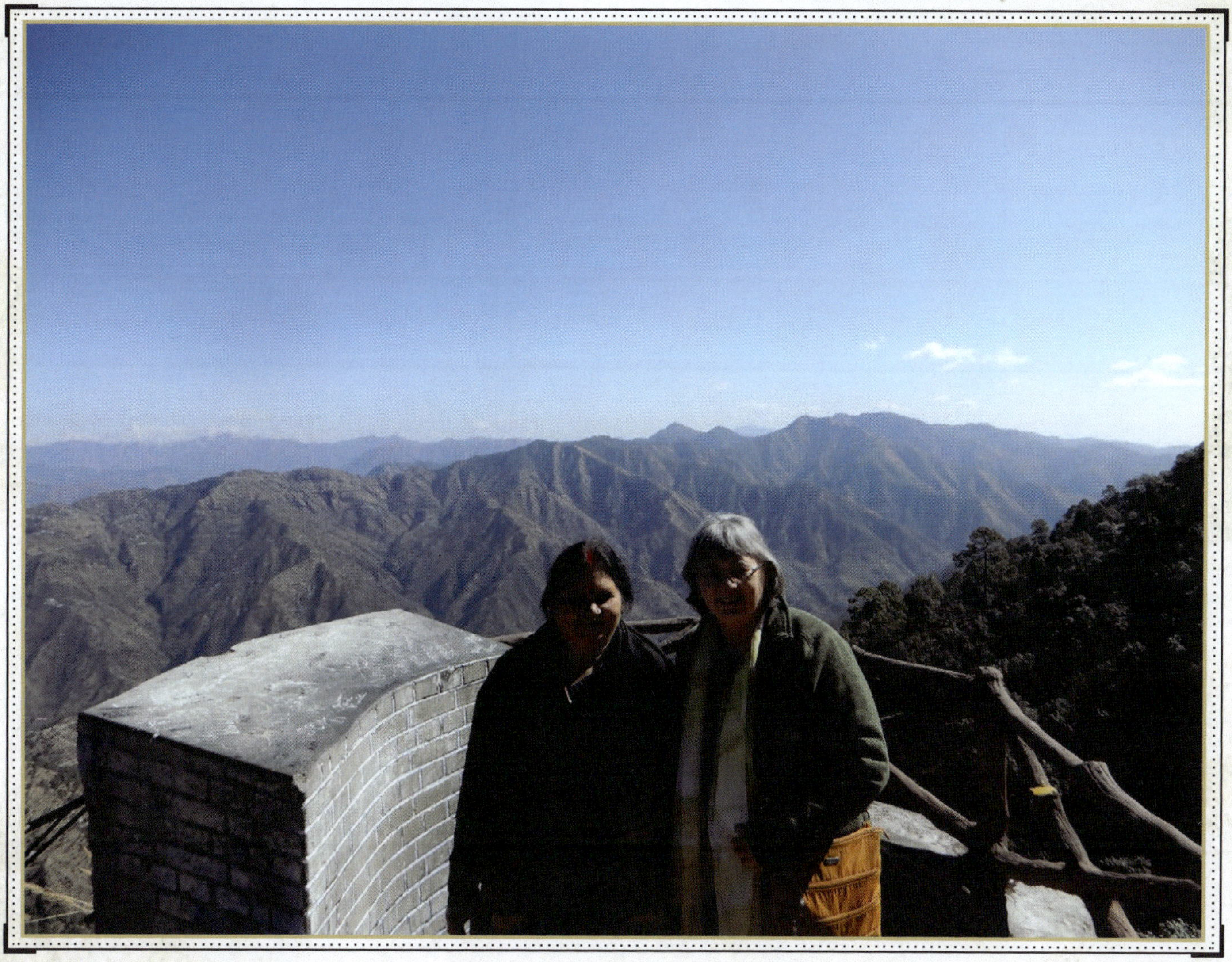

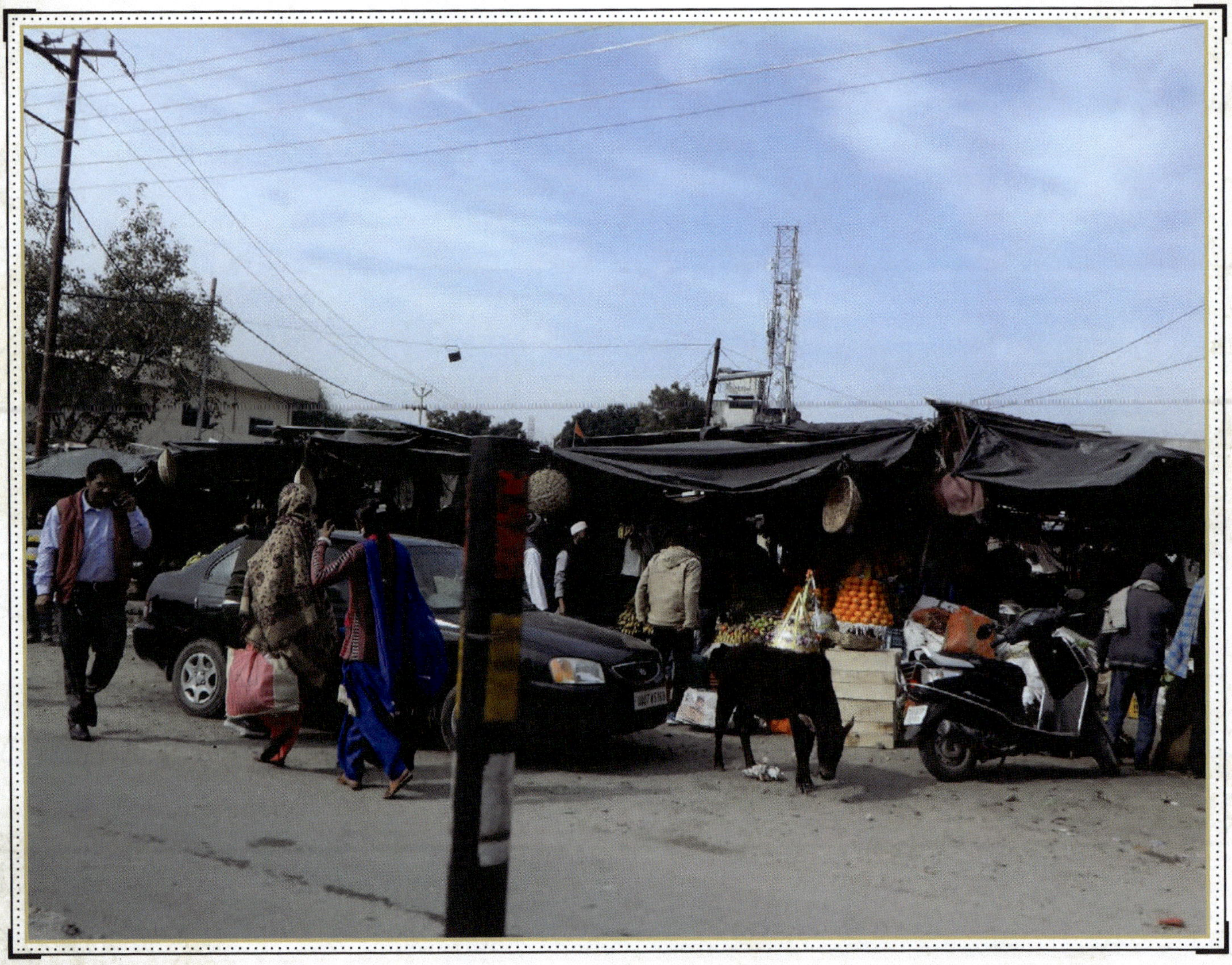

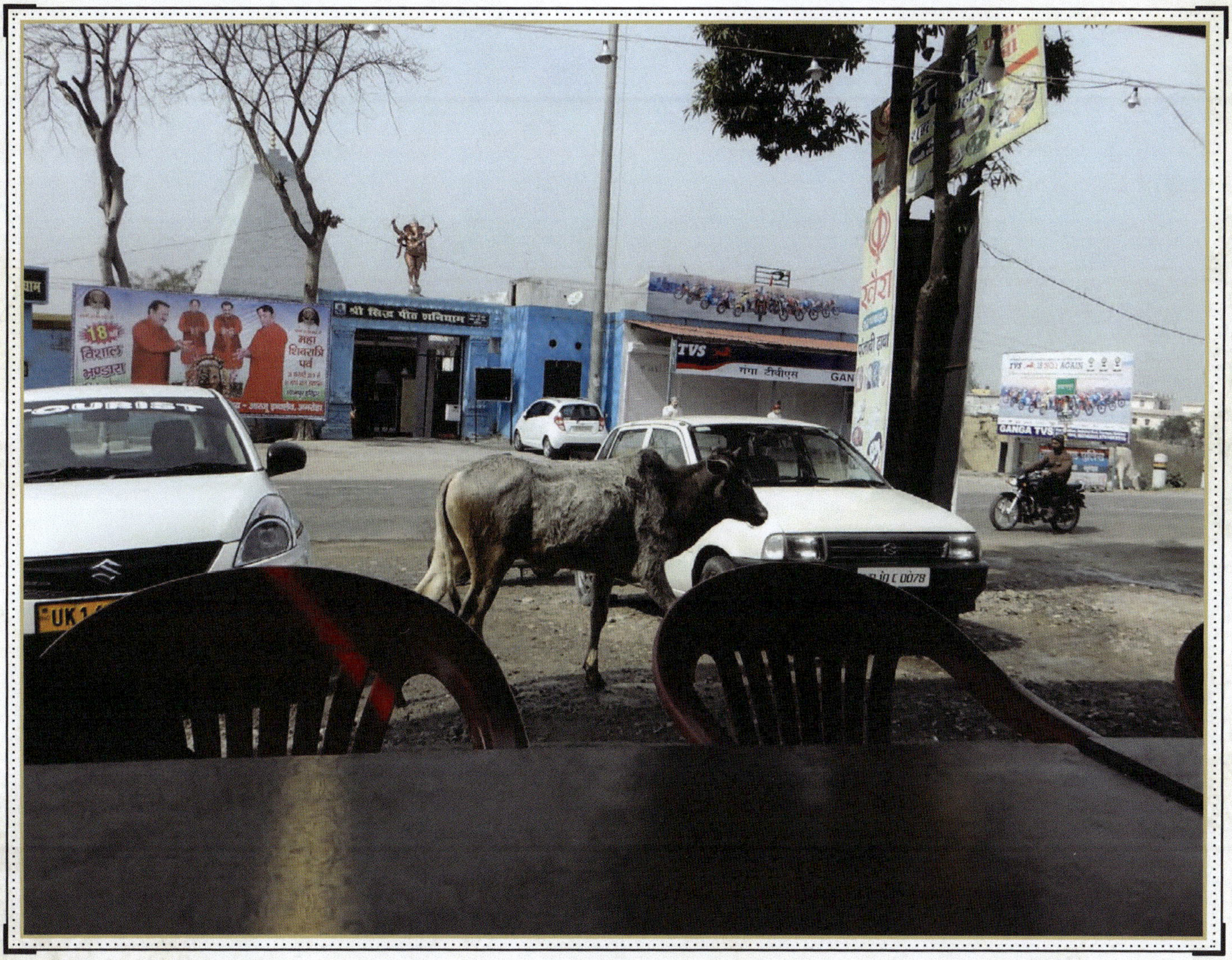

18
विशाल
भण्डारा
महा
शिवरात्रि
पर्व
TOURIST
TVS
गंगा टीवीएस
GANGA TVS

Day 14 and 15

(Haridwar)

The days in Haridwar are like a dream. Here a drop of the elixir of immortality spilled over accidently from a kumbha pitcher being carried by the celestial Garuda bird during the ancient churning of the ocean of milk which created the world. I am concurrently reading "Autobiography of a Yogi". The quest for spirituality in his early days is running parallel to my visit to this ancient domain of human spirituality. I am writing this recollection of my first two days here at a comfortable table on the guest terrace which is located just outside my spacious room. Here at the Haveli Hari Ganga hotel, you live like a queen in an oasis of comfort with central heating. The hotel is small and luxurious. The terrace abuts right up against a tributary of Ganges River which then meets again the Ganges further downstream. As I write this, I can see the fast-flowing water and on the opposite bank about 200 feet away is a quiet park where people sit and then go bathe in the river.

It is quite amazing to be so close to this energy source. Santosh and I have walked twice to the sacred Aarti ceremony held in the evening as dusk falls. It is held at the Har Ki Pauri (footsteps of the Lord) ghat. It is greatly meaningful and enjoyable to listen to the devotional hymns chanted by seven priests, hear the old and very large metal bells rhythmically struck, and see the flames lit at the end of the ceremony. As we sit close to the banks of the Ganga, small flames float past us on green leaves, placed in the water by family members.

Last night, I closed my eyes in meditation during the ceremony, and a vision of the Divine Mother came to me in infinite white and brightness. It is so wonderful to be travelling with Santosh who is, himself, very spiritual and able to explain the rituals and the history of India, and who is himself devoted to the sacred. Yesterday, we went up a sacred mountain by cable car to visit a temple at the top. It was suddenly so peaceful; we could hear birds singing and we watched the pilgrims below us who had chosen to walk up the steep terrain.

On the hotel patio by the river, I have my palms read by an expert palm reader and Vedic astrologer, Mr. Bhaskar Yogi. He is quite young, perhaps late 20's or early 30's and has been taught by his father and grandfather in these arts.

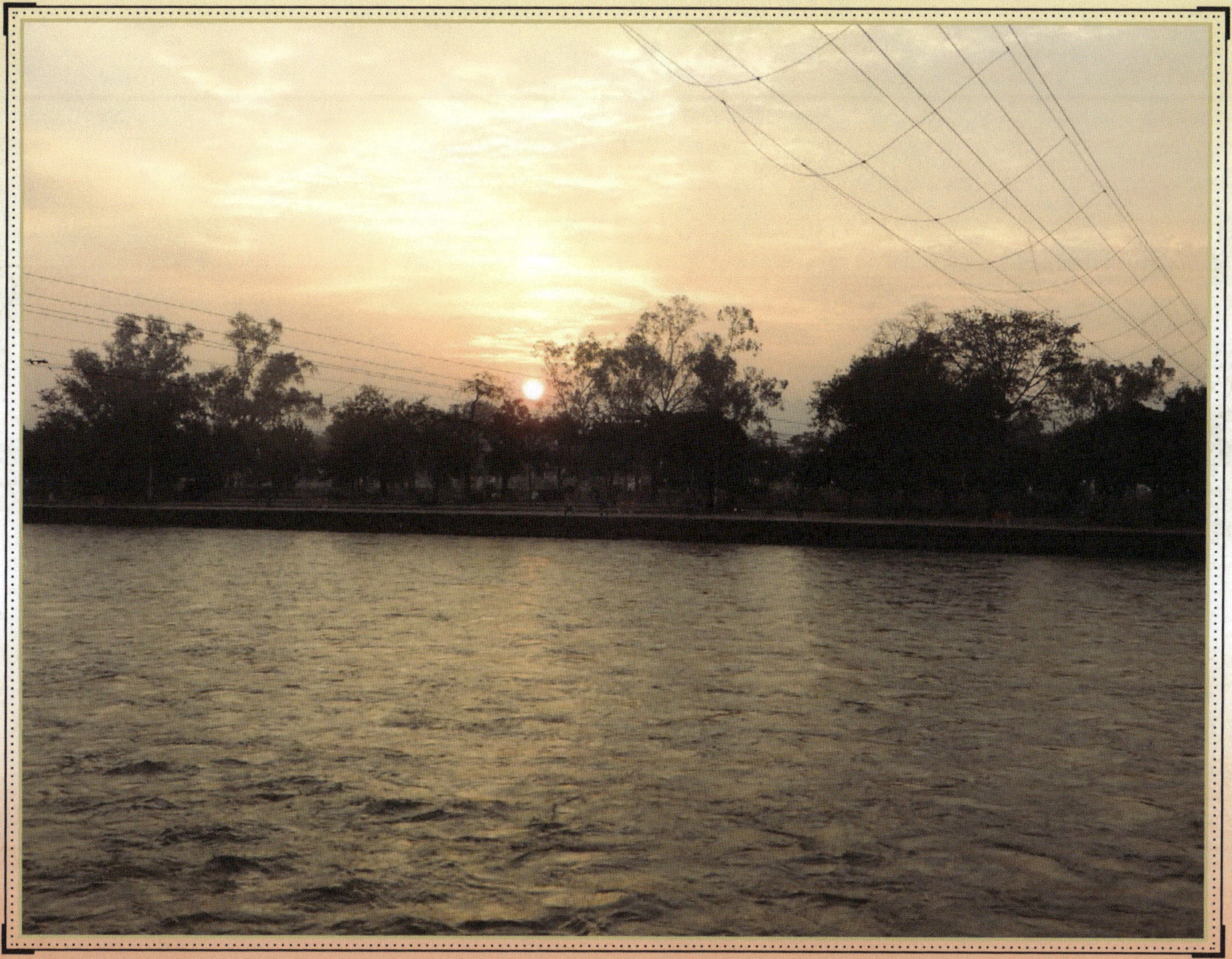

My hands show the planet Jupiter and I know immediately that he is accurate because my Western astrology rising sign is Sagittarius ruled by Jupiter. He says "get ready" for lots of travel. He repeats this twice. He says I worry about my fulfillment; I am not totally satisfied although life is smooth, and that by May 2019 things will come together more clearly. He says I was close to my Dad but he was taken too soon. He says I came from nothing and through hard work, I have achieved everything (so true.) I am surrounded by good friends who support me. My health is good in life and I will be healthy and active to the end of my life at around 90 years old. If I survive a bump at 90, I can go onto 95. I am independent by nature. I have a good and open heart and am honest to people. However, I can be too outspoken at times. "Get ready, ma'am, for travel" he says again. I tell him I have Ashwini Star and Moon in Aries, and so does he, and he may help me to learn Vedic astrology. It is so amazing to be seated directly by the flowing Goddess Ganga listening to this very learned Vedic astrologer.

Although I am engrossed in the direct experience of India, tears still fill my eyes at the thought of Kelly. He is still so big a part of my identity as a soul. Last night at the Aarti with the flowing river current at my feet, I remembered when I had placed Kelly's ashes into Shawnigan Creek which flowed through our property. They were still warm as I had, in devotion, stood outside the small countryside crematorium, and watched the smoke rise which was his body disintegrating into air. I received the warm ashes in a jar and placed them into the car and, when home, walked around the property with them and then I walked directly down to the creek having also retrieved the ashes of his beloved golden retriever, Charley, which Kelly had kept by his bedside for ten years. I placed both sets of ashes into the stream together and watched as the milky white ashes merged with the fast-flowing stream water. It is a strange moment that.

I still do not understand this world or this phase of life. But I know I am free now, wherever that takes me. In the earliest days after his passing, Kelly came to me in voice three times calling my name with such a joyful quality. And he has appeared in dreams, and in spirit readings to say that he is happy and is busy. I am sure a lot of this trip is his doing. His wish for me is to be happy and live with joy!

Day 16

(Haridwar)

A beautiful leisurely day just walking around the busy markets. I am more used to the sudden blaring horn and step adroitly to the left. The markets are full of brass pots and colorful shawls. These shawls are not of the fine woven threads of the Kausani shawls. I have asked online if I can buy the luxurious Kausani shawls elsewhere other than Kausani but they appear to be sold only locally to that area. We spend the day, Santosh and I, on the river's edge watching the many people of Hindu faith taking their holy dip and thereby receiving blessings from the Goddess Ganga. Men and women, especially in family groups, clasp tightly to the metal chain fence as the river here narrows slightly and increases in current. Sometimes we observe deities being taken to the river with lots of excited chanting and happiness. We spend more than two hours just sitting and absorbing. Santosh has taken his holy dip early in the morning at sunrise with some friends made at the hostel where he is staying. In the evening, we watch again the Aarti ceremony from the opposite bank, listening again, for the third day, to the beautiful devotional chanting of the priests, and watching again the glorious fire ceremony with hypnotic ringing of ancient bells.

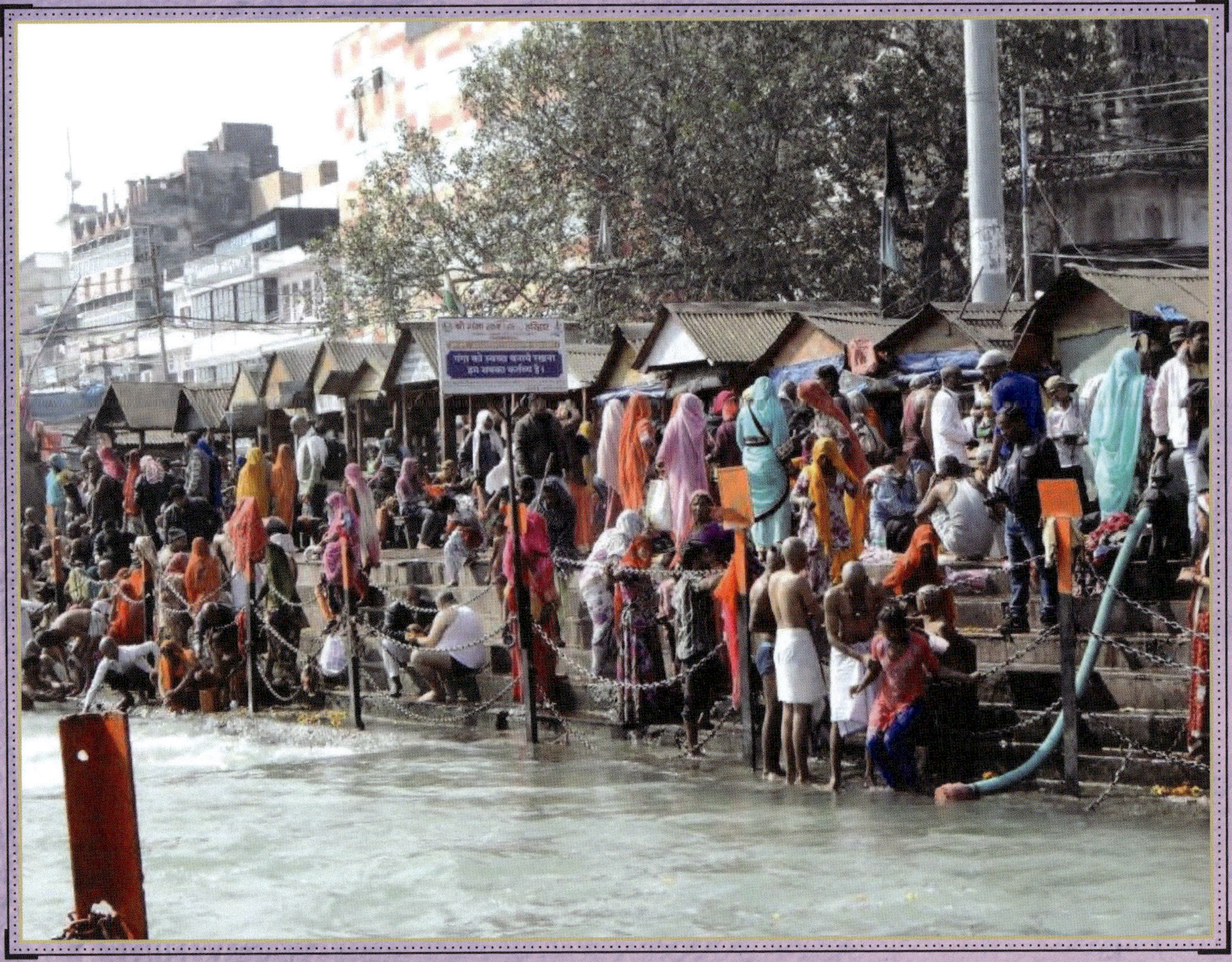

The Sweet Flowing Goddess Mother Ganga

All along the sweet flowing Goddess Mother Ganga
Holy bathers seek unity
With the sacred waters of Heaven

At sunset, the pulse is deepened by
deep devotional mantra
Time worn, eternal bells ringing
Reminding us of an ancient home

Fire in our hands
Burning into our souls

Goddess Mother Ganga
We sing and pray to you

Goddess Mother Ganga
Your flow in my veins
Takes me to God

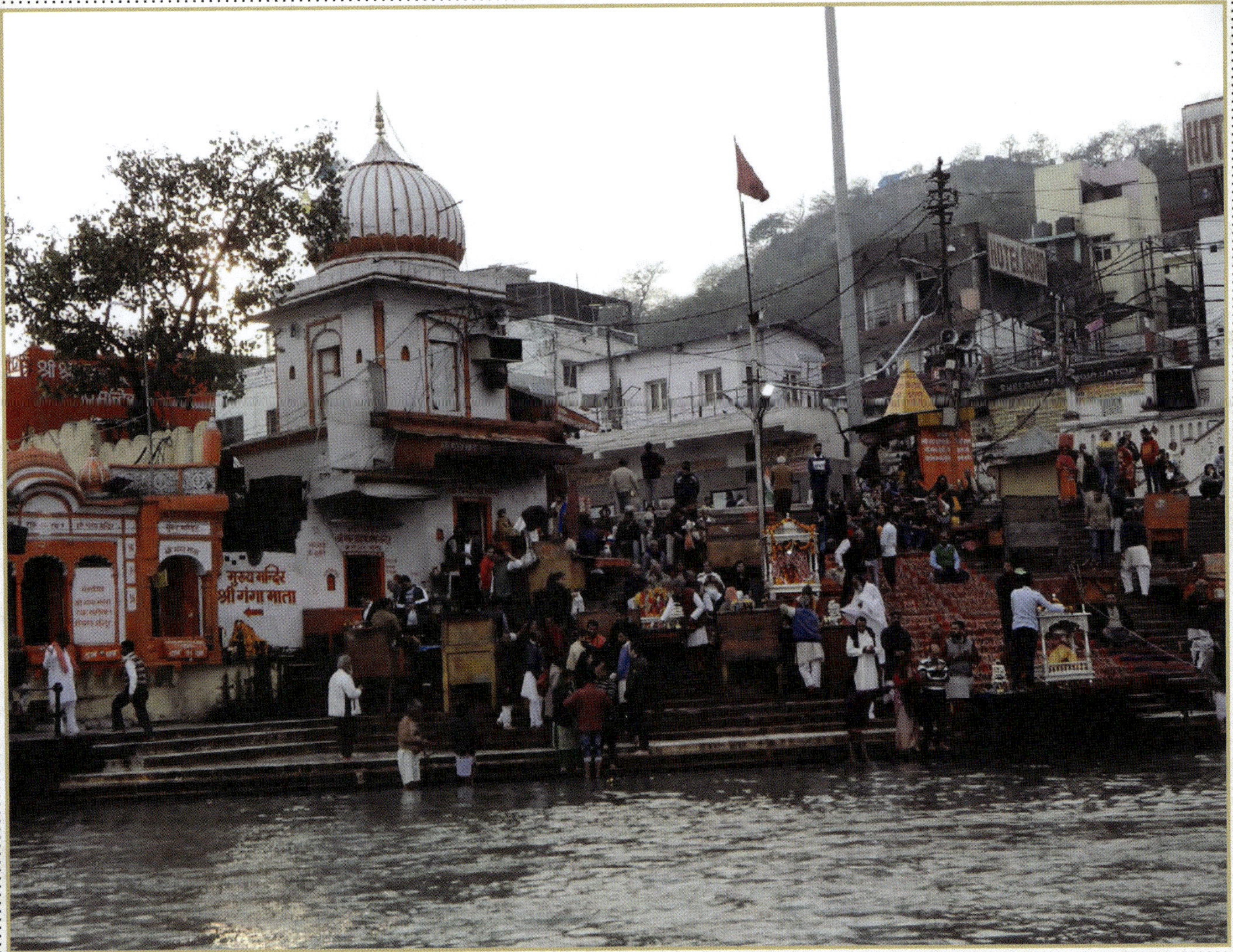
मुख्य मन्दिर
श्री गंगा माता

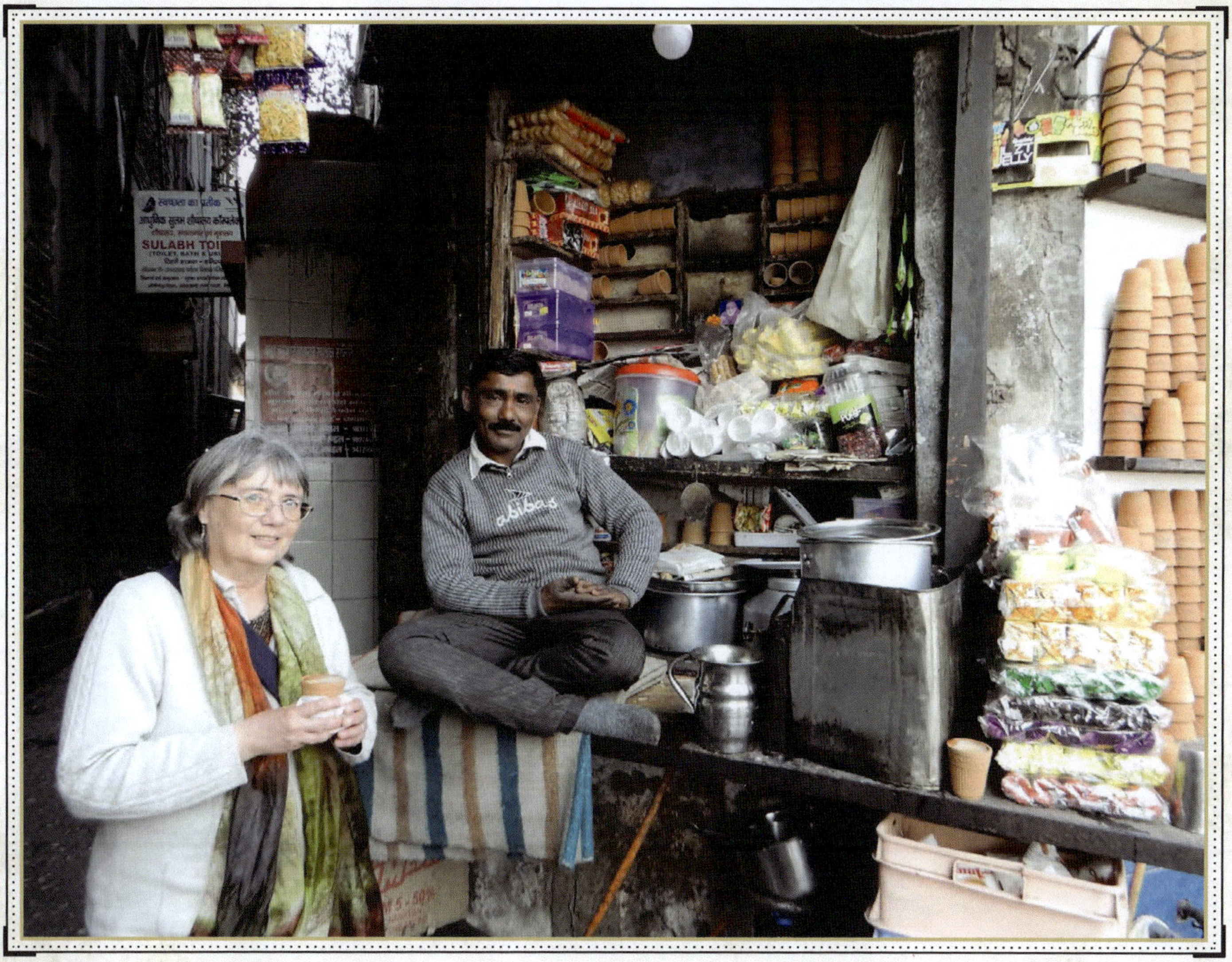
SULABH

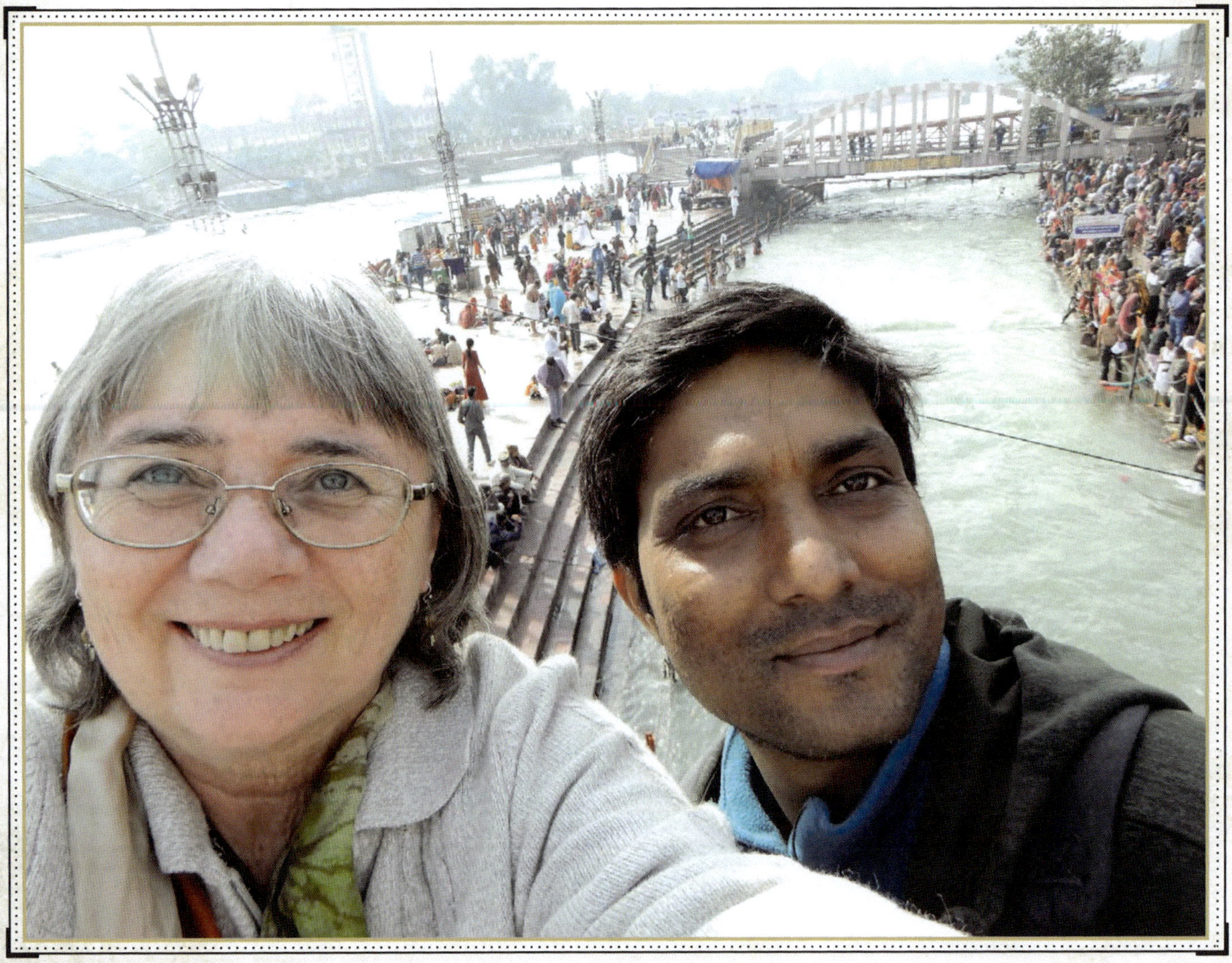

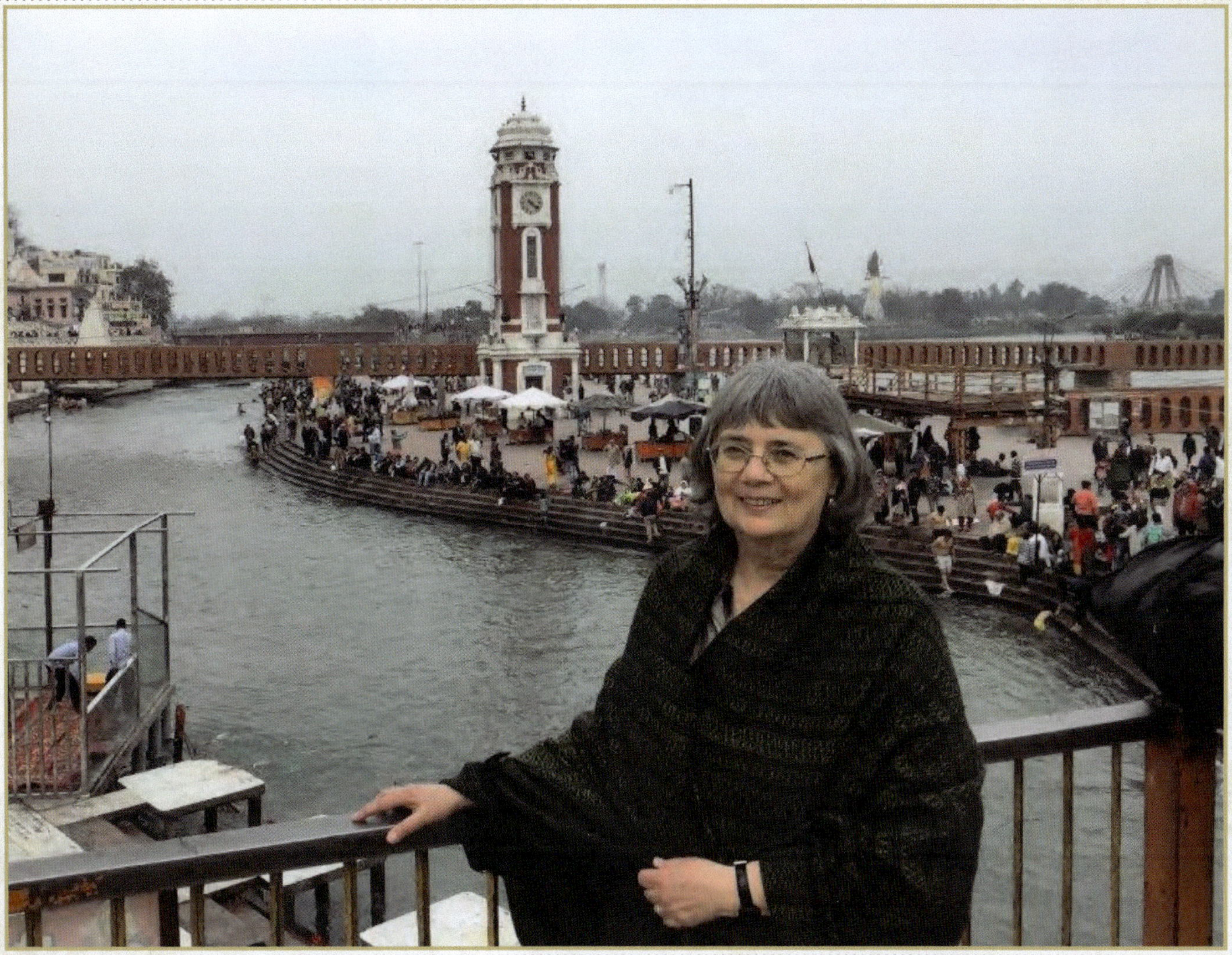

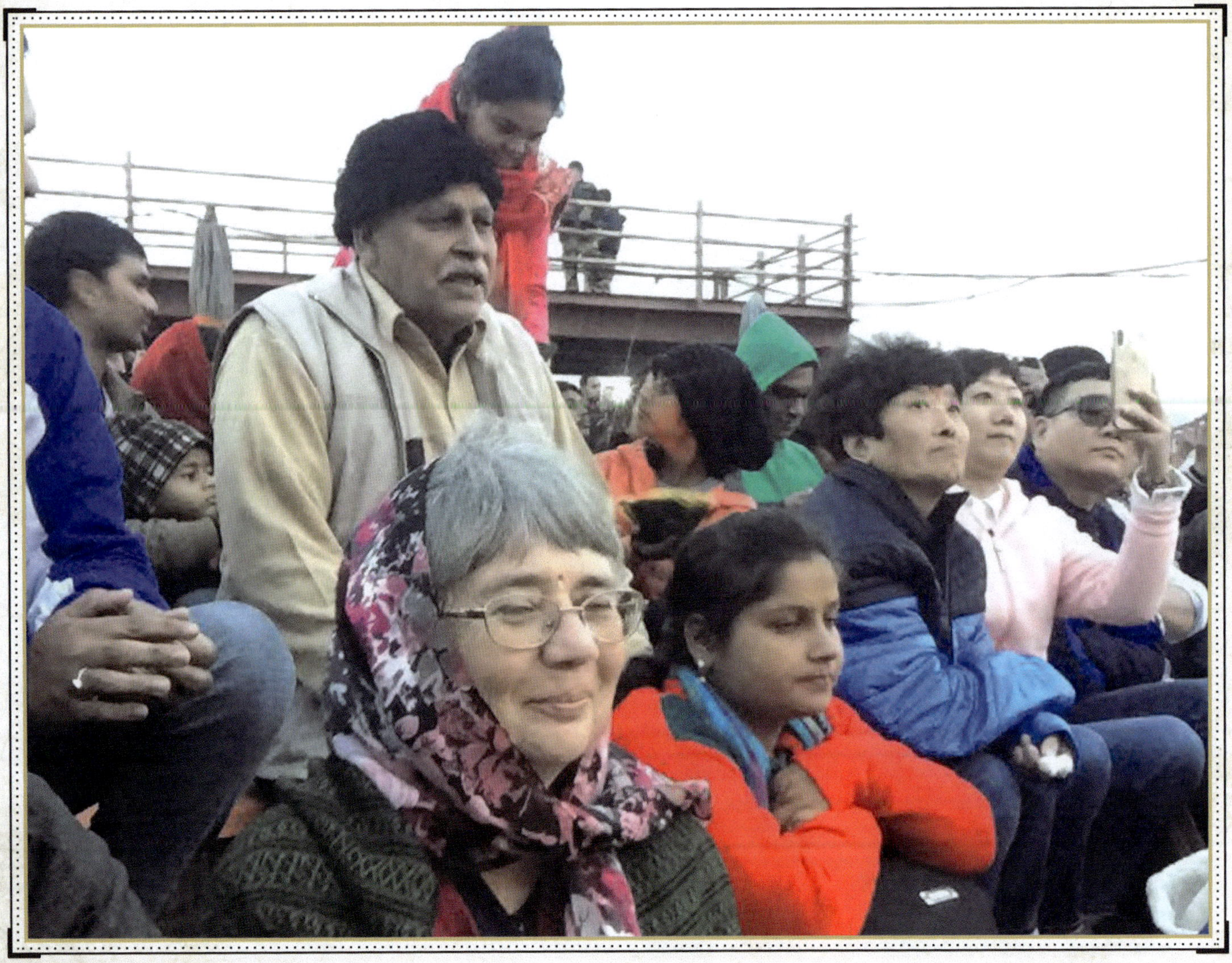

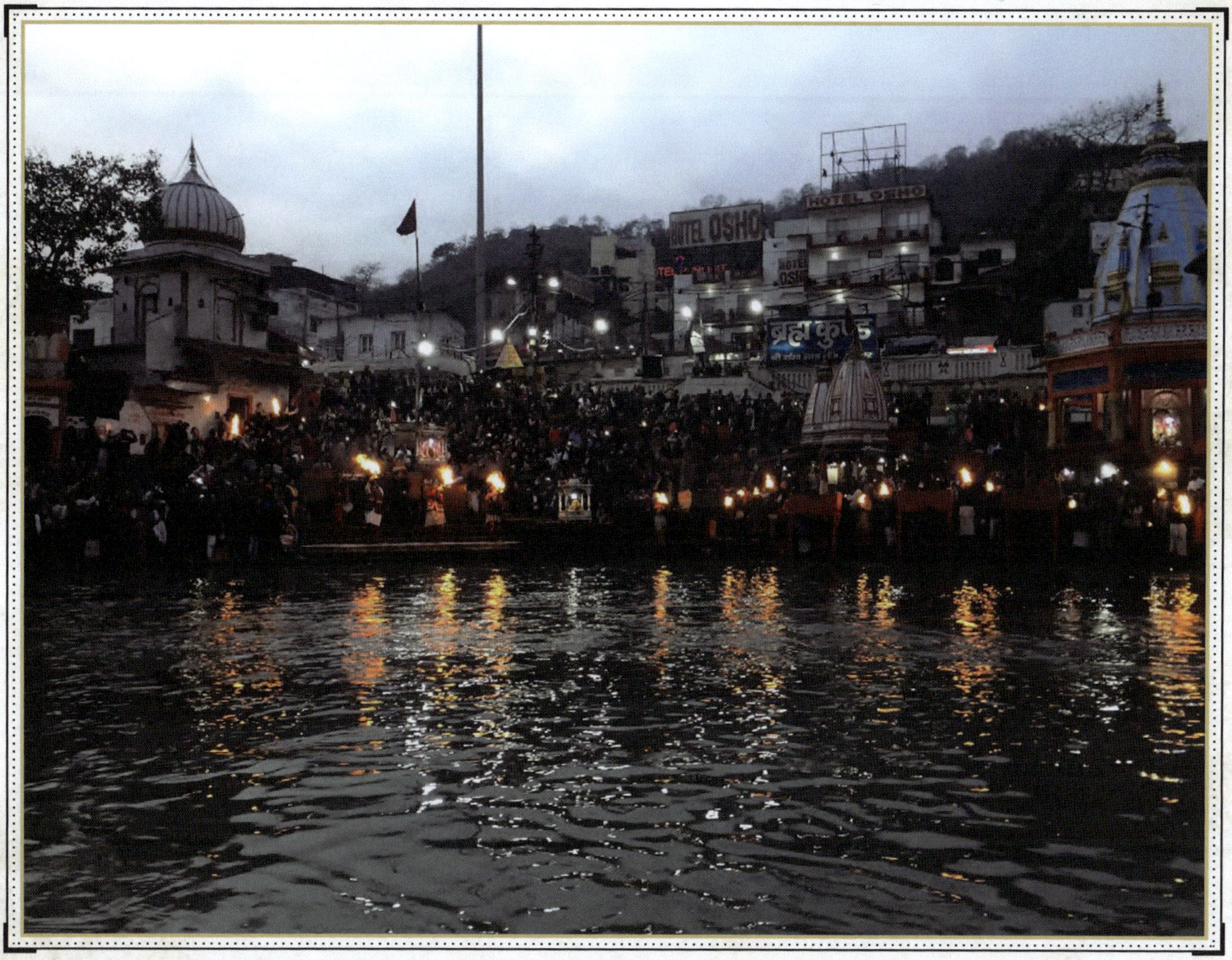
HOTEL OSHO

Day 17
(Haridwar to Srinigar)

My dreams again are of Kelly and that he has taken a new partner, one with pigtails, and I must divorce him and divvy up the property into half, and try to make a new life. I think again this is only my mental processing of my new reality and his. This is very hard work and part of my healing process of grief. I have no answers. My Vedic astrologer said yesterday that Kelly is a good person and that God likes to surround himself with good people which is why Kelly is with God and happy.

The road to Srinigar is long and winding with heavy traffic due to train crossing stops. We stop at a most beautiful place, however, where the Alaknanda River and the Bhagirathi River converge near the town of Devprayag (Godly Confluence.) The physical convergence of these two rivers becomes the River Ganga but it is also known spiritually as the Goddess Ganga and Mother Ganga. It is said the Lord Vishnu accidentally poked a hole into the universe with his toe, creating a place for the Goddess to flow over his toe and flow uncontrollably from heaven onto earth. Lord Shiva who is symbolically all the snowy high Himalayan mountains was petitioned then by the Goddess to capture the water through his many dreadlocks of hair to prevent damage from such an onslaught of high water.

Santosh and I walk across a suspension bridge over the Bhagirathi River. The bridge has a few lounging cows who are very calm and friendly, and then at the far end, a group of happy school children come toward us and pass us on their way home. On the other side, we walk on stony steps through a small village and bazaar with small shops, and then down into a temple area by the water convergence. This is a holy area and several bathers are there. I give a donation to a priest who insists on my repeating various Hindu mantras, and once he has gone, I do some personal meditation. The one river is deep and deceptively calm; the other is quick and active with small rapids. A couple next to us asks for pictures and we have a lovely photo shoot. Then Santosh and I climb back up and, on the way through the small bazaar area, I notice beautiful black beads and pick up a set. They will always remind me of this beautiful moment with the Goddess Ganga.

We carry on to the hotel which has a stunning view of the Ganges River. However, some services are very lacking, and I can tell the standards and the food are really low in quality so I decide against dinner. A few hours later, a knock is at my door and I do not answer as I am not expecting anyone and I do not want to answer as a female. The knocking continues and a voice says "room service", however, I have not ordered anything. He keeps trying the door to come in, but as always, I have the upper bolt on. I do not answer and instead phone the front desk for them to check it out. Eventually, the situation is resolved and he retires but it has made me realize again how much easier it is to travel with a companion.

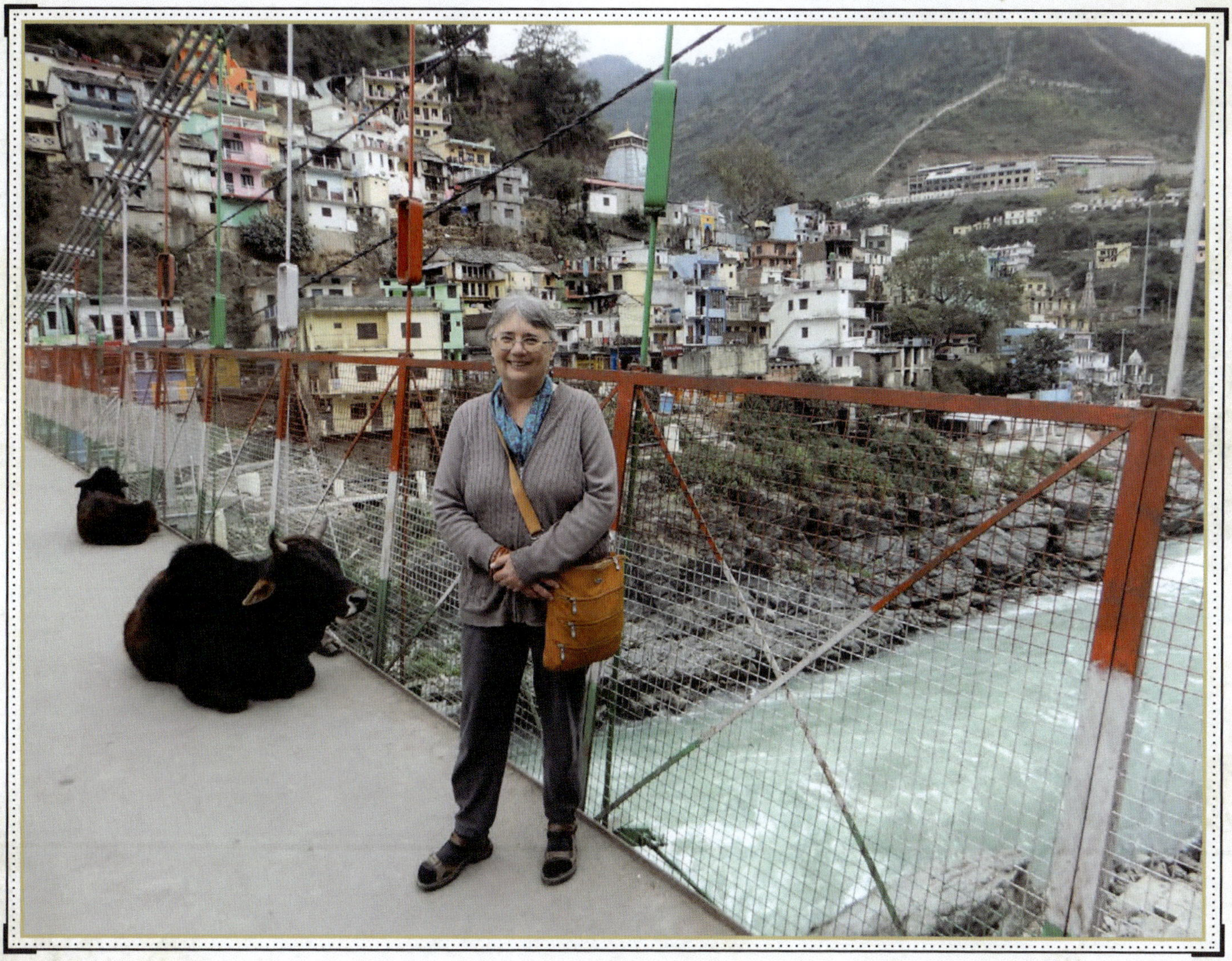

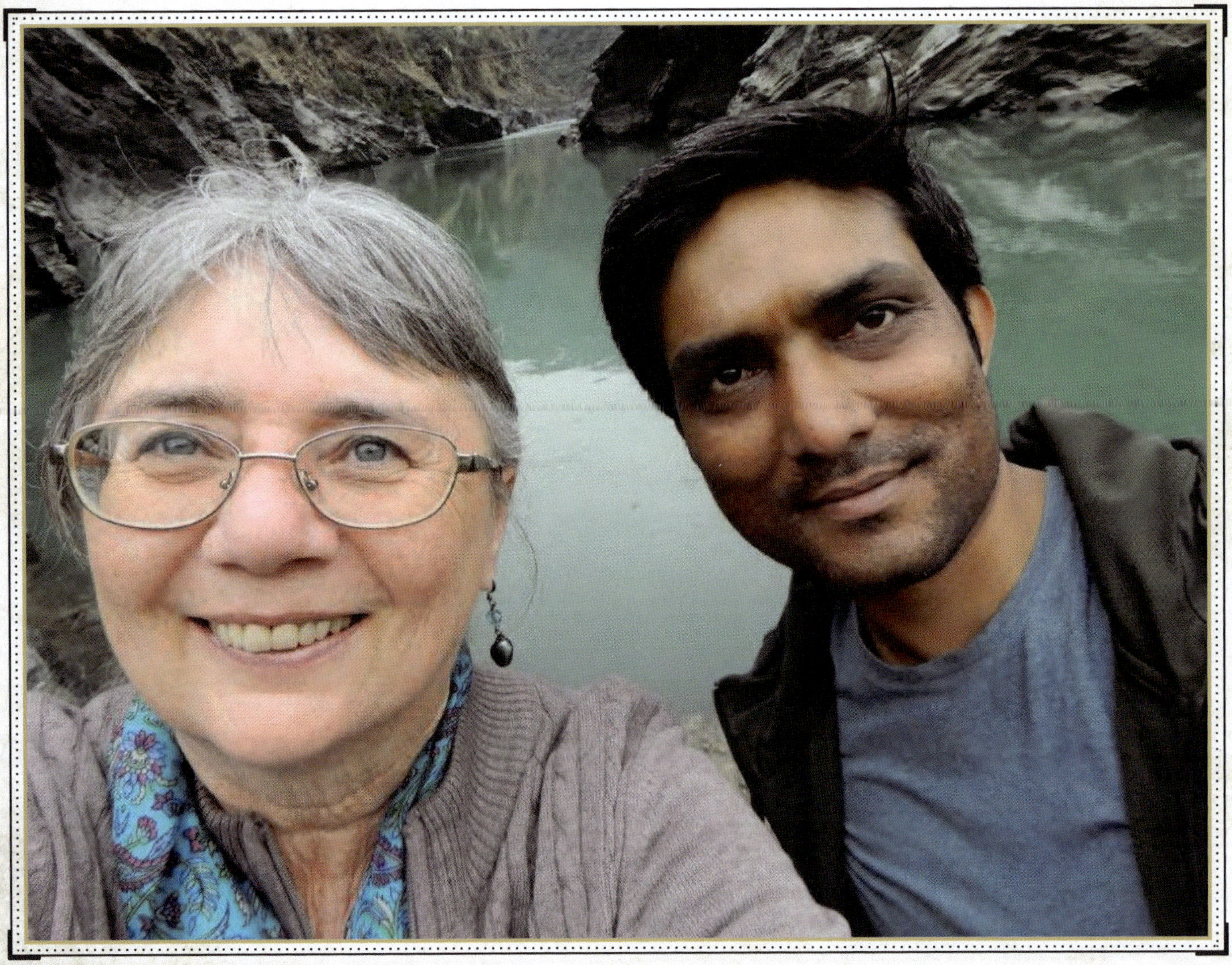

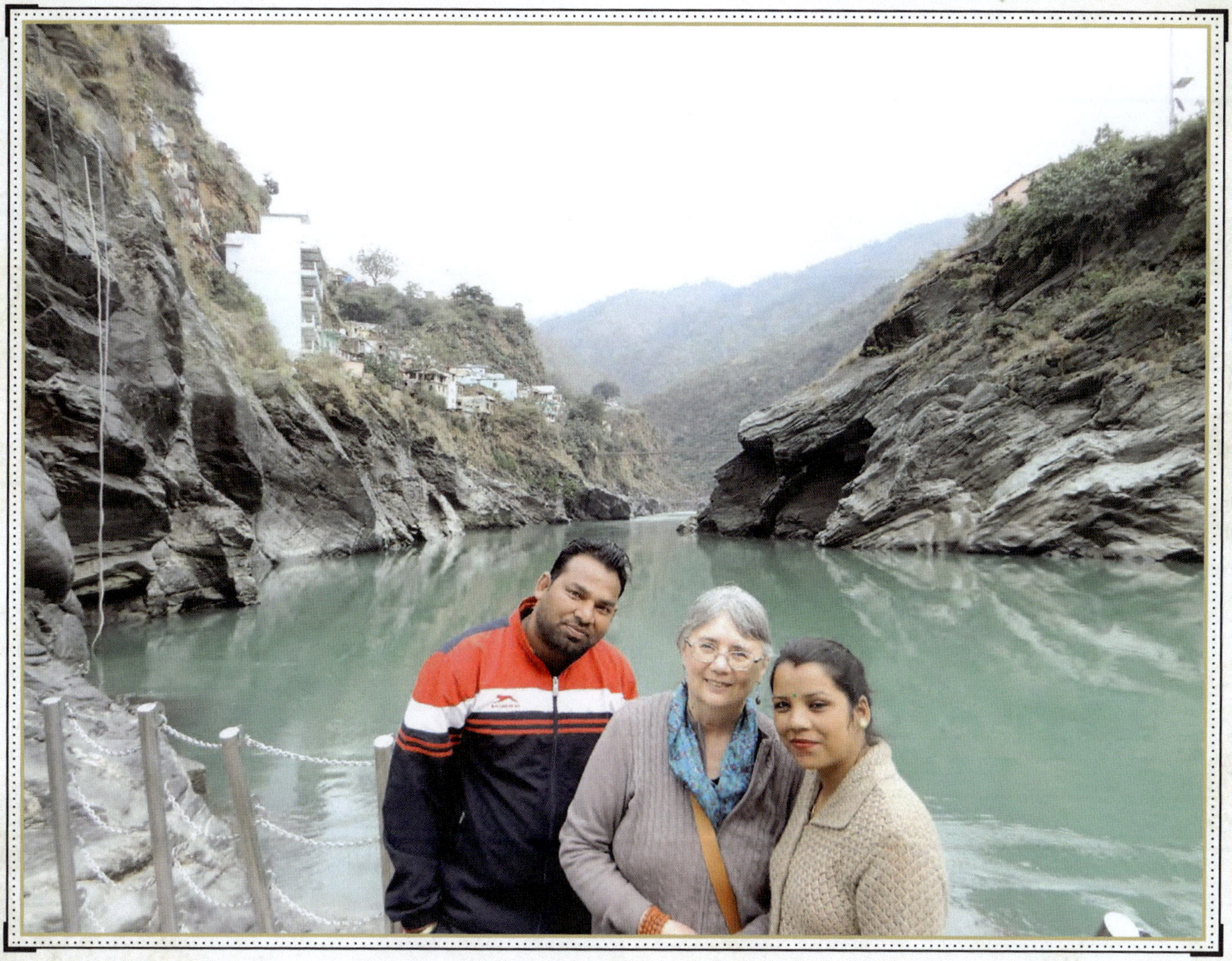

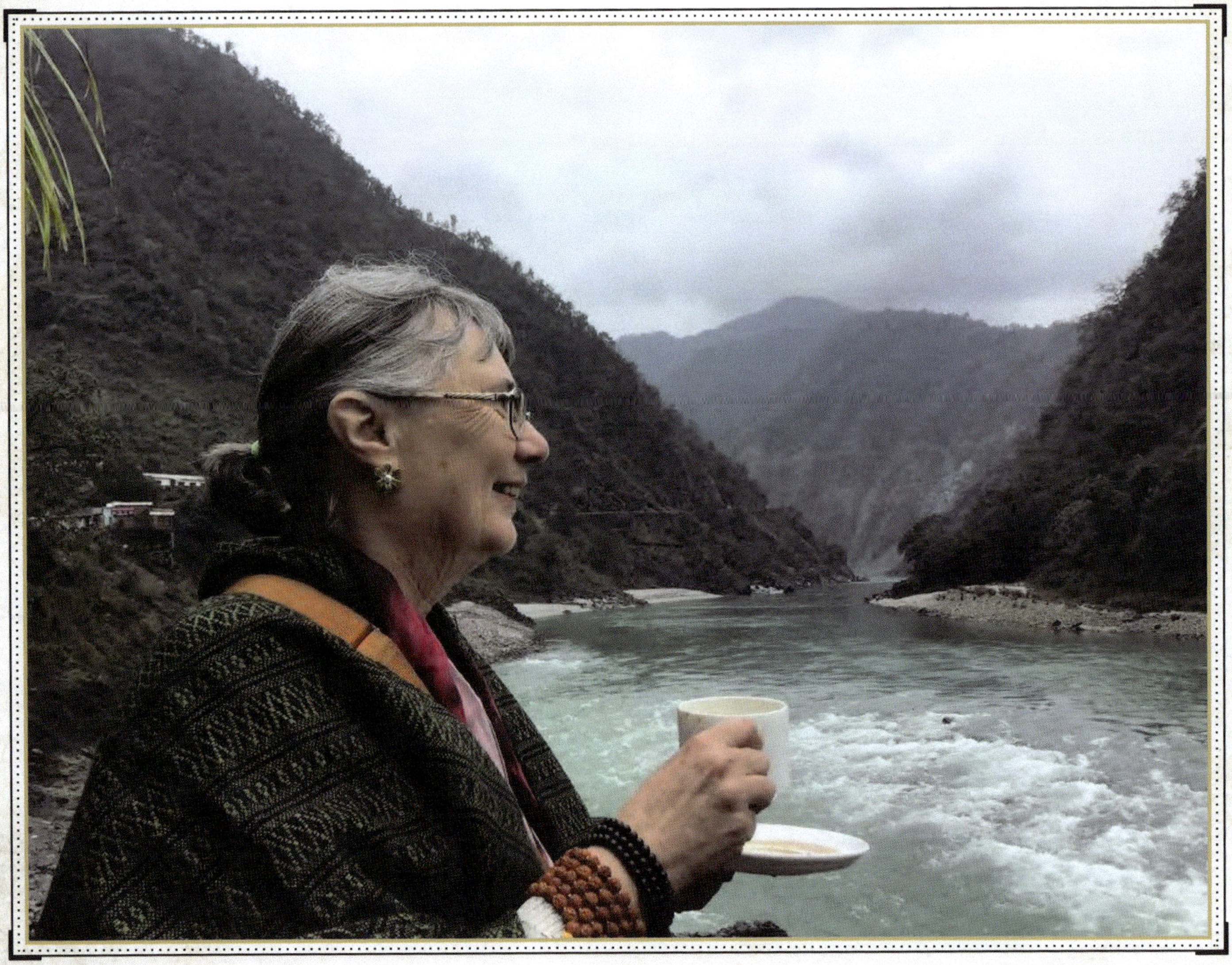

Day 18

(Srinigar to Rishikesh)

Early in the morning, I head out onto the balcony and do ten rounds (10 x 108 beads of the mala) of the Shiva mantra "Om Namah Shivaya". The balcony has a stunning and close proximity to the Ganges River. Last night, after seeing the weather reports of continuous heavy rain and also feeling my energy much lower, I made the big decision to skip this mountain range of Gurwhal and instead go to Rishikesh for an extra five days. I had phoned Santosh and, as usual, he is completely on my side. Unfortunately, I will not see Shiva in his mountain home on this trip but this is only a reason to come back for another try.

We begin our journey back down the mountain pass in absolute pouring rain, another omen that my decision to reverse my plans was good. Today is Valentine's Day, and even though Kelly and I never celebrated Valentine's Day, instead treating every day as a "love" day, I am momentarily overwhelmed with my loss. Our last Valentine's Day was in India in 2017 at the Golden Temple in Amritsar where Kelly bought me a stuffed red heart-shaped pillow to celebrate. He was gone the following January.

We stop at a local restaurant at the river's bend. I had seen the restaurant from a distance and knew instinctively the feng-shui (good vibes) was incredible. I have always been good at knowing which is a good place to eat! I head down to the Ganga River's edge and Santosh shortly brings down chai from the restaurant. What a glorious experience. The air and river feel vital and fresh. Again, many photos are taken.

Finally, we embark again and I am taken to the Hotel Natraj, a modern hotel in Rishikesh, with many conveniences. I rest briefly and at 4:30 pm, Santosh and the driver and I head to a local market next to the water's edge. Many sadhus abound. Lightning and thunder and finally more rain appears as we sip chai under an old tree. It is a lovely finish to the day.

Day 19

(Rishikesh)

A good breakfast to start the day. I sit next to a whole group from Israel all saying "Shalom" to each other in the hotel dining room. After breakfast, Santosh picks me up and takes me through a tourist market that is next to the Ram Jhula bridge which we cross to the other side. Motorcycles and people all share this swinging bridge and I have learned to step left whenever I hear a horn. On the other side, we walk through another small market area which turns into a street of ashrams where international students can study yoga and meditation. We turn into the Parmarth Niketan ashram with its spacious courtyard. After enjoying its peaceful environment, we cross the street and go down to the water's edge where a wedding canopy is being prepared in front of a beautiful Shiva statue. The wedding party is small and well-dressed and I think they must be from the ashram to be able to have this intimate and meaningful wedding in this location so close to the Goddess Ganga.

I sit on stone steps away from the wedding party and closer to the water, along with Santosh on a different level of step and a meditating priest on a flat area a few steps above me. I see a dog coming with a purpose towards me and then the lovely, gentle and delicate female dog comes directly to me to say hello with a nudge of her head delicately on my arms. We share a moment and she sleeps on the step above me. Santosh brings me water from the sacred Ganga in his hands. The wedding ceremony has begun with bride, groom, priests, and about twenty family members. After about twenty minutes of watching respectfully at a distance, we keep walking down the street and then loop back to the Parmarth Niketan ashram and indulge in a delicious thali-style lunch from their canteen, including naan, dahl, spinach with corn, and rice. No excessive spice or onions or garlic is used in the preparation. As a special treat, Santosh has ordered each of us a gulab jamin which is a deep-fried flour ball soaked in honey. It is back across the Ram Jhula bridge the way we came and back to the hotel for me to get a couple of hours rest.

At 4:30 pm, Santosh and Gajendra pick me up and off we head again. The storm with heavy monsoon rain has returned so Aarti is out of the question. Instead, we drive to a good local restaurant just for a chai. The rain stops but it is still too wet for walking with large puddles everywhere so we drive along a canal that is an offshoot of the Ganga and which waters local farms. Finally, it is back to the hotel.

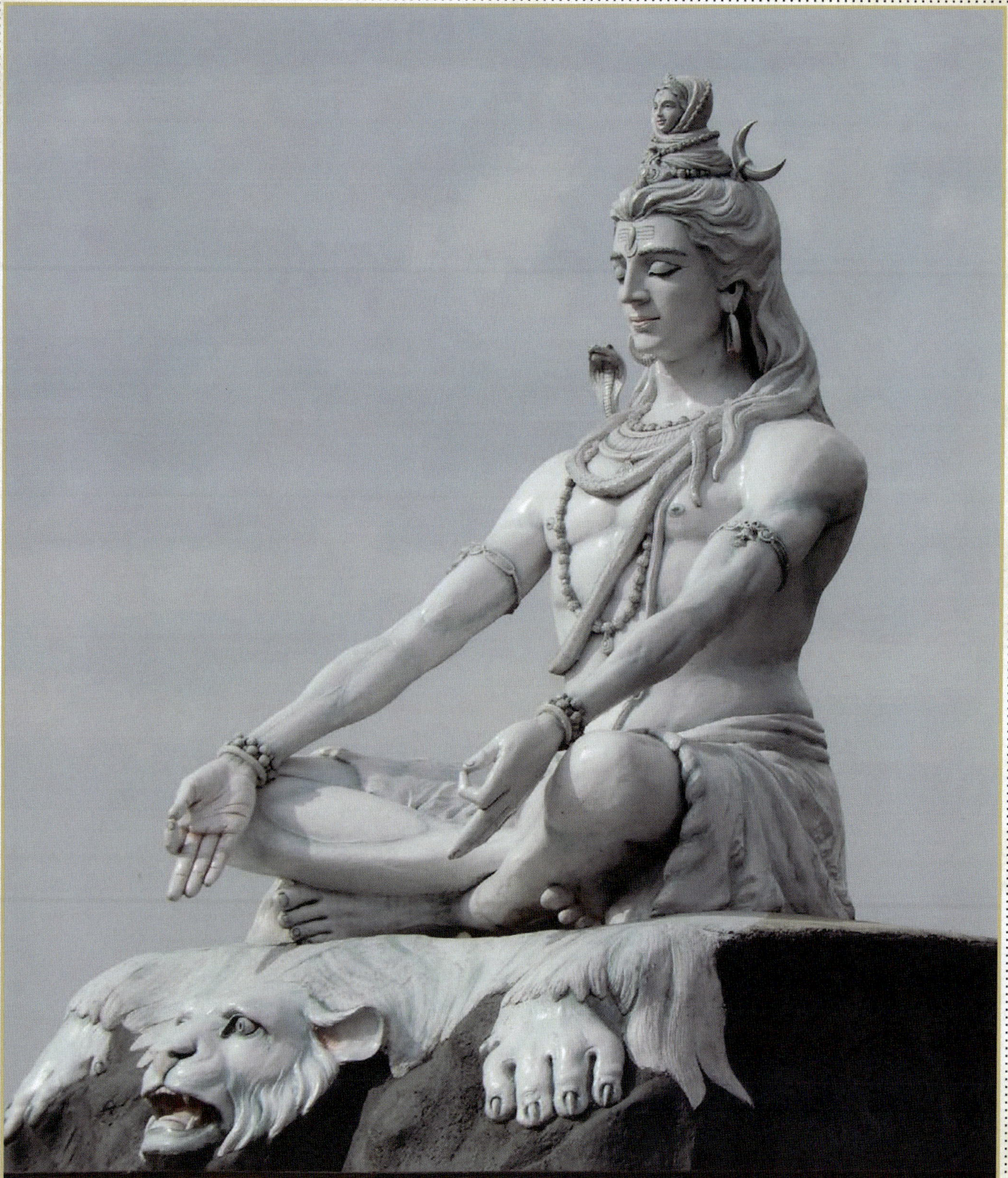

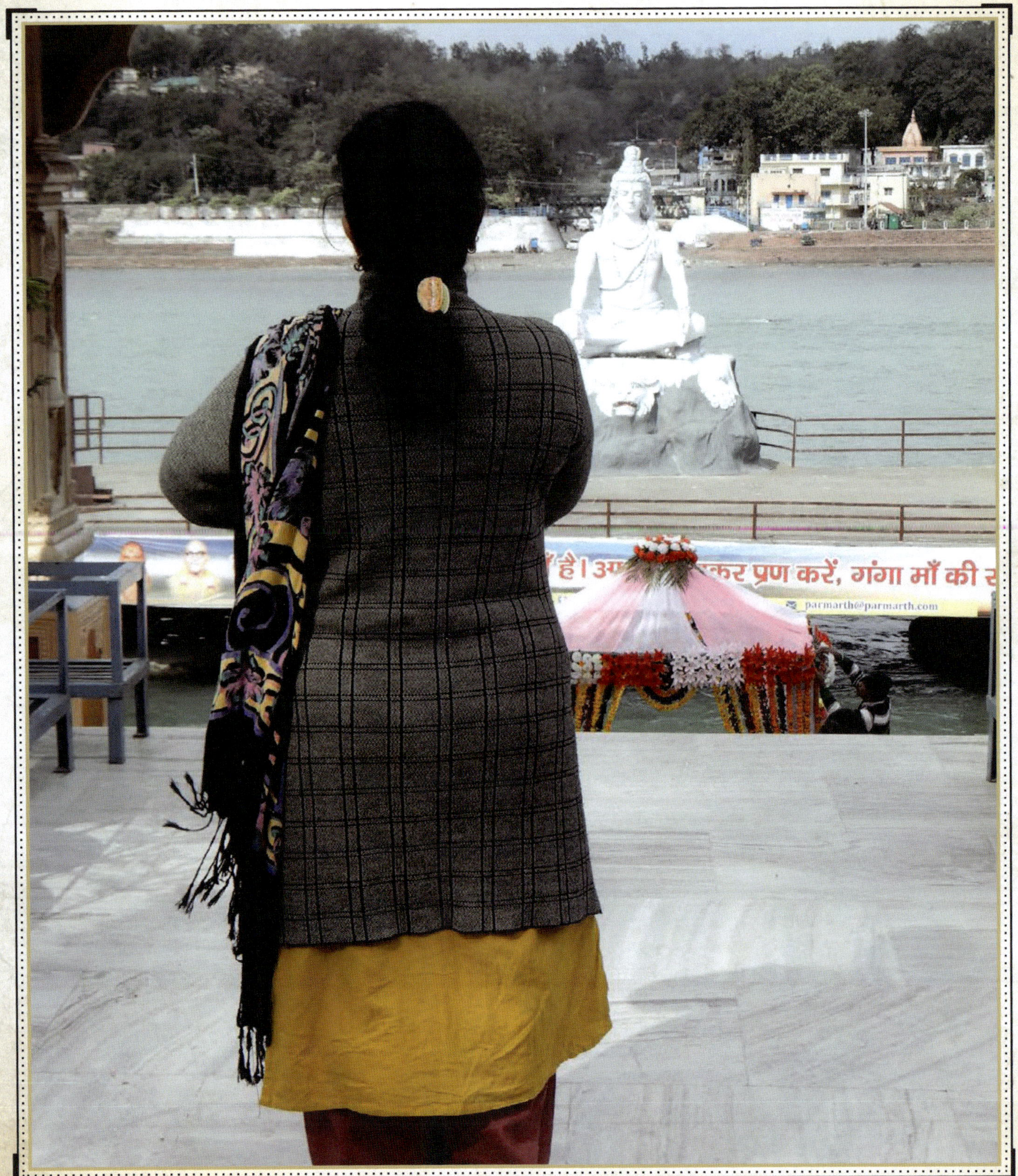
प्रण करें, गंगा माँ की
parmarth@parmarth.com

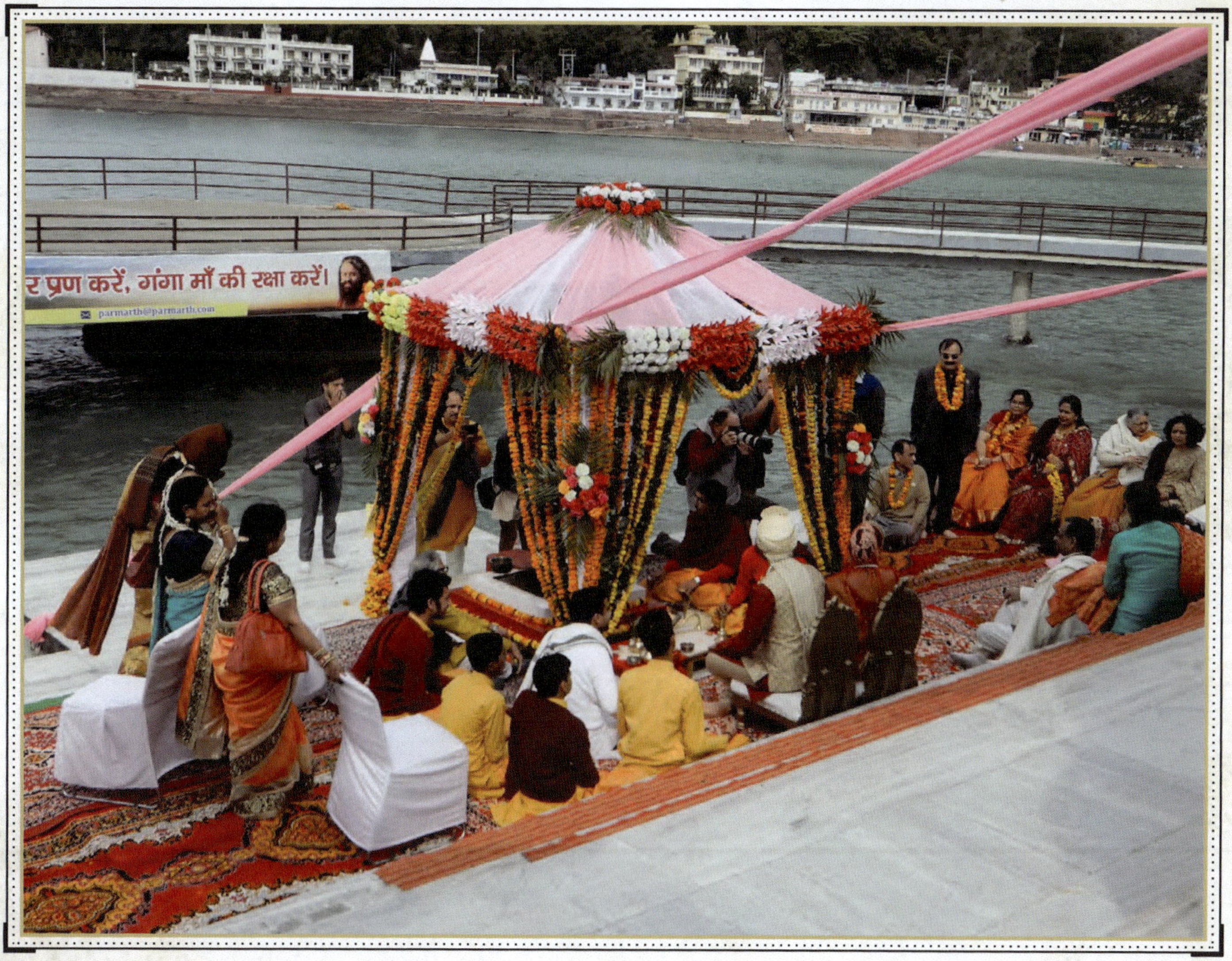
र प्रण करें, गंगा माँ की रक्षा करें।
parmarth@parmarth.com

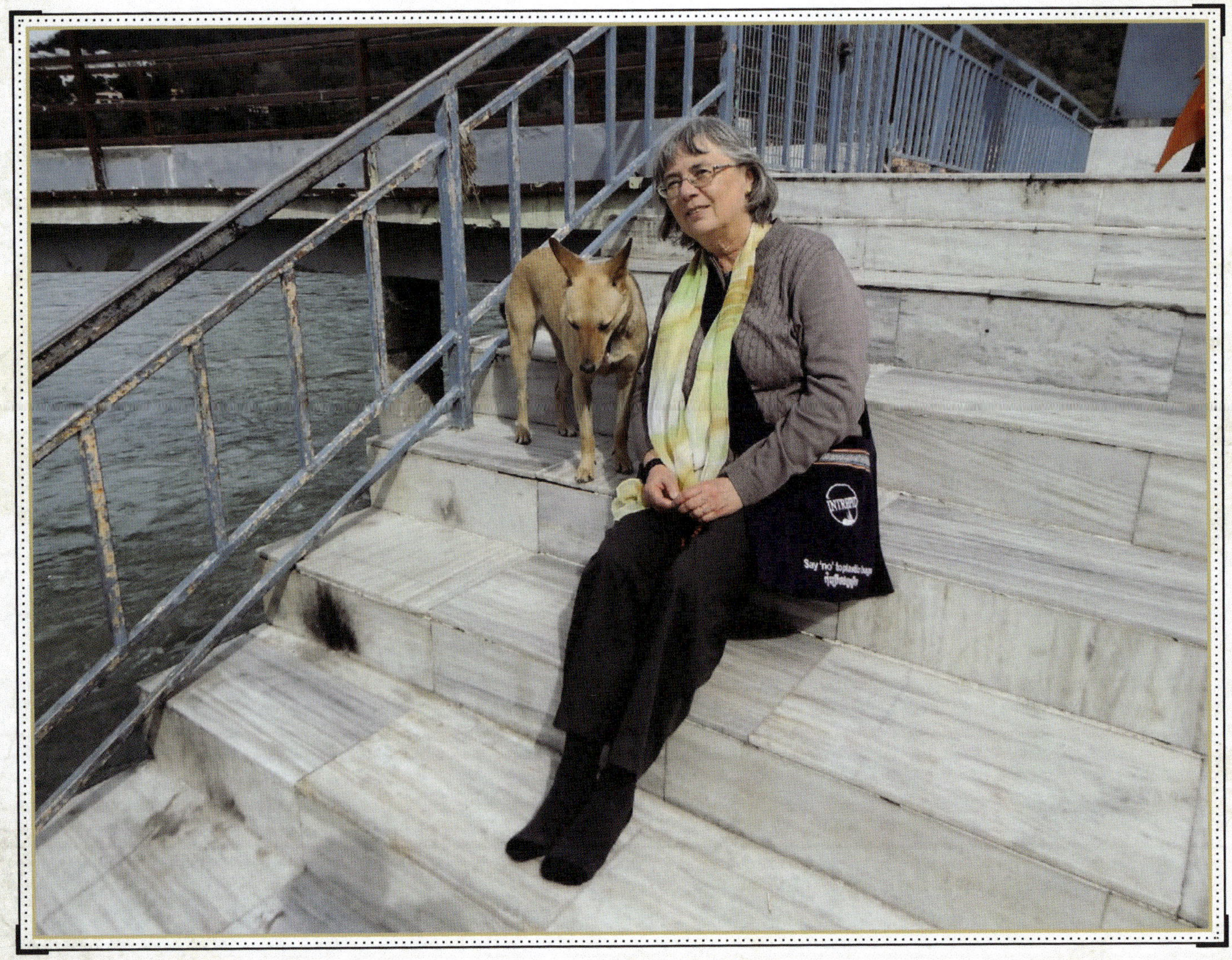

Day 20

(Rishikesh)

Today, we again cross the Ram Jhula bridge but turn left and down to a sandy area by the Ganges River. I sit on a boulder and contemplate the flowing water. There is a small group of sadhus on the opposite side. In a quiet moment, I settle my mind to try to understand how I am feeling. I generate light and warmth from within. Then the meditation is over and Santosh takes some lovely pictures of me against the Ganga backdrop. He tells me he has taken a holy bath here before. We turn up to the road and go back to the area of the Parmarth Niketan ashram along this narrow country lane which is nonetheless filled with cows, people, goats, motorcycles and sadhus. We reach the end of the road and because I have a sore throat, Santosh kindly orders lemon and hot water with added raw ginger and honey. It is a delicious drink and I tell him that on yoga retreats in my teen years, I had used this drink for fasting but with black pepper also added. I meet a young gentleman from Japan who has been to Vancouver where I grew up and to Whistler. He carries a small tambourine which he expertly plays as he walks away. Santosh and I take a side street to the ashram and he has a solid good lunch but I am not hungry and I only have gulab jamin again.

After lunch, we take a passenger boat, which fits about thirty people, on the way back to the other side of the river. Two young Western men join in the rousing Indian mantra choruses of a Mumbai women's group. They have the whole boat singing and clapping. I take a break in the hotel until 4:30 pm and, this time, Santosh and I take the boat first, to cross back to the ashram side for Aarti. We reach the ashram ghat and choose seats close to the musicians. This Aarti is all self-sung and the music indescribably moves through my whole body.

A devout group of South Korean young women cluster around the fire offering area in a circle and offer devotional prayers. The whole ceremony is about one hour long and incredibly beautiful. At its end, Santosh and I go back to the same shop for hot lemon juice and ginger. Walking back, we pass a small hermit-like cell where several sadhus are gathered singing devotional prayers. Then it is off to the bridge but there is a black-out in the area including shops on both sides and including the bridge. But this does not mean that the oncoming motorcycles slow down. I am very grateful when we get across the bridge safely and the lights go on halfway through the market.

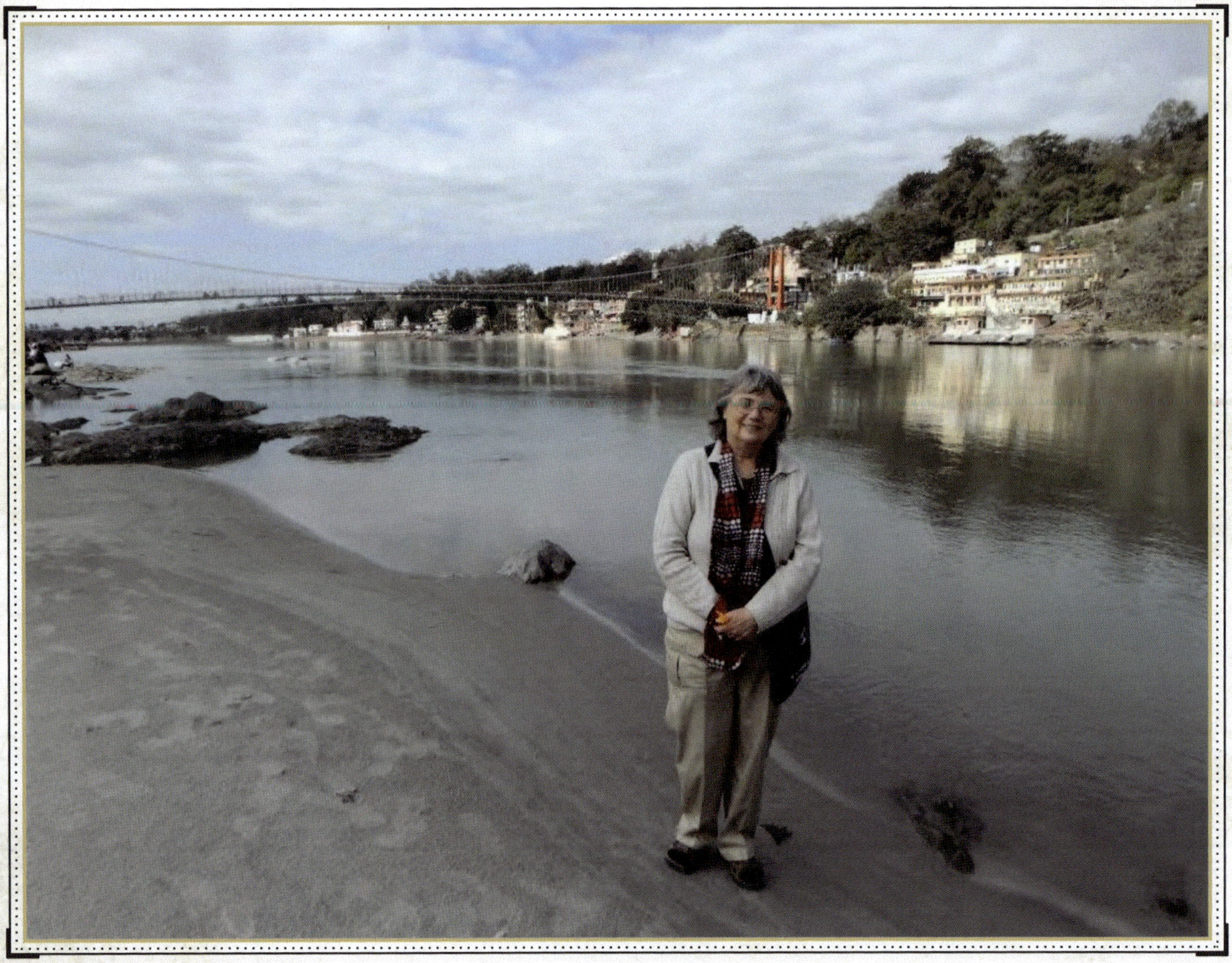

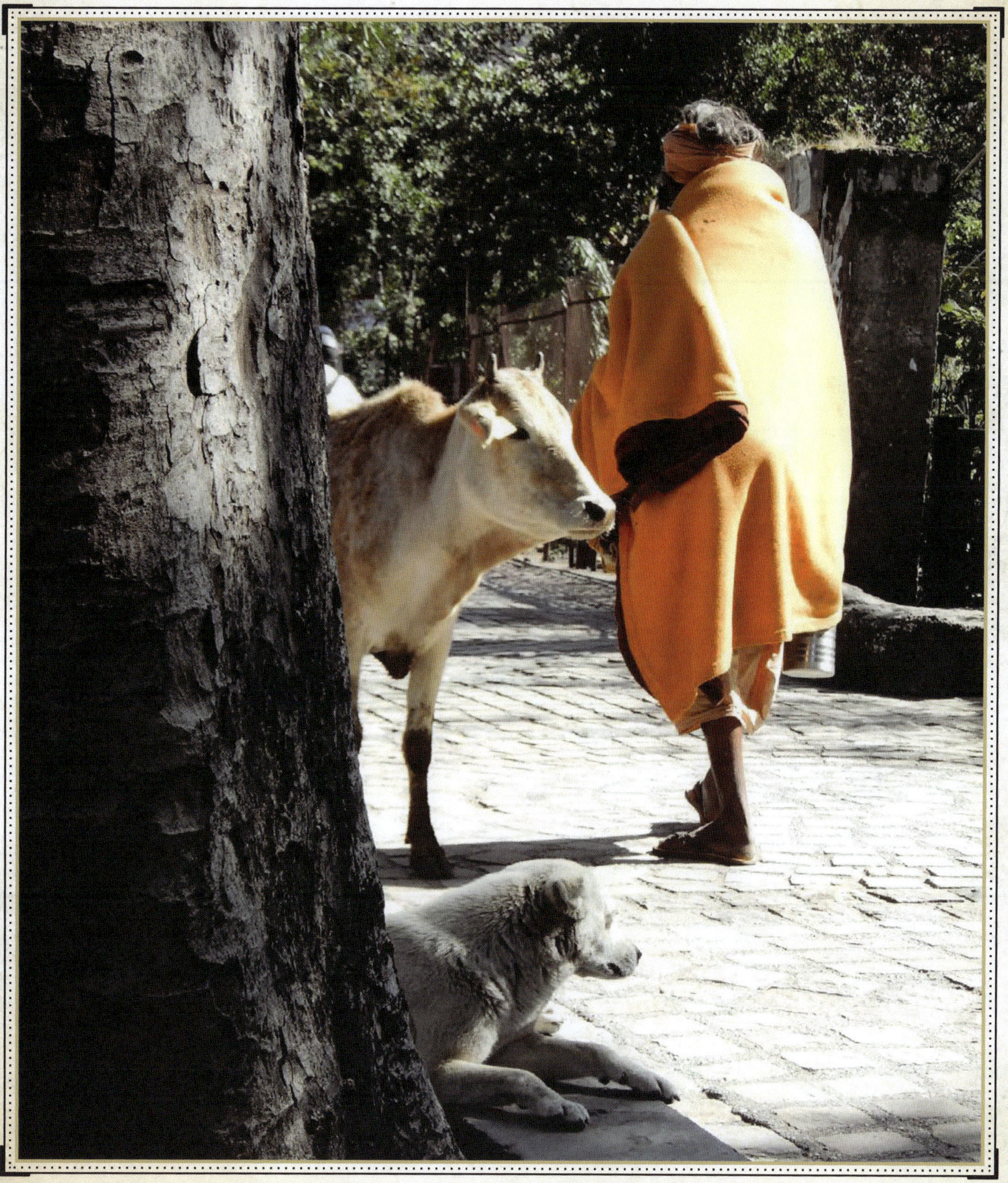

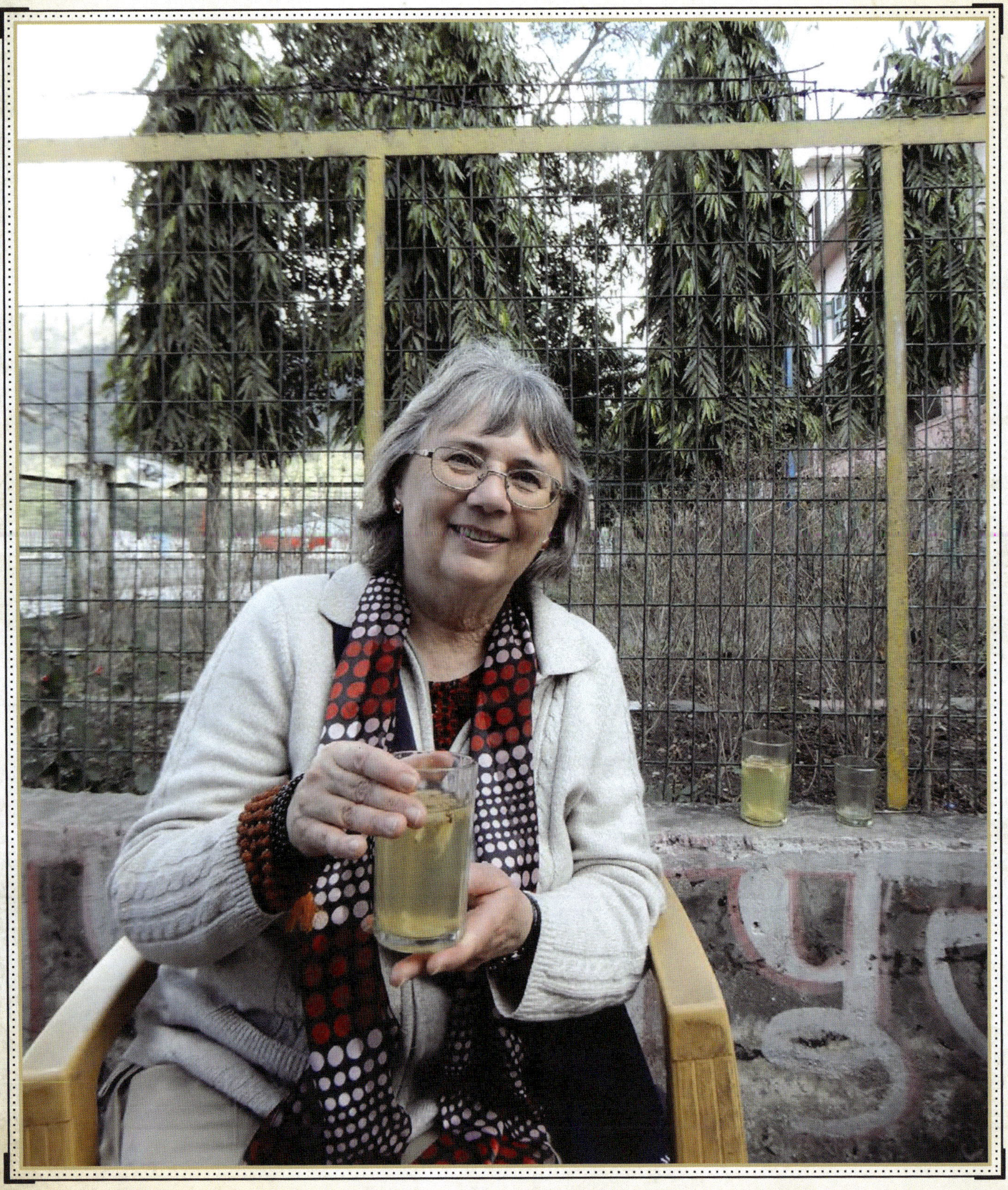

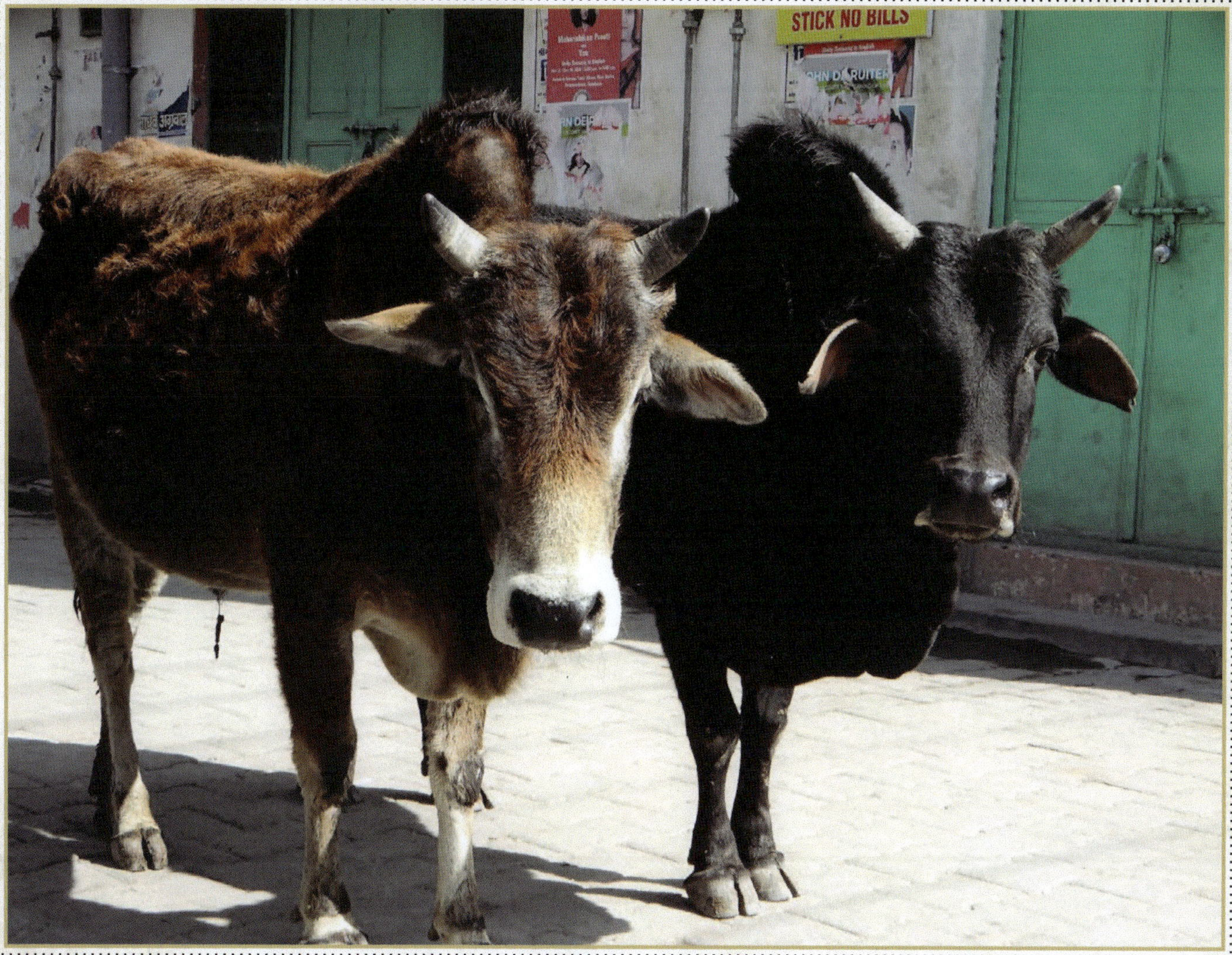
STICK NO BILLS

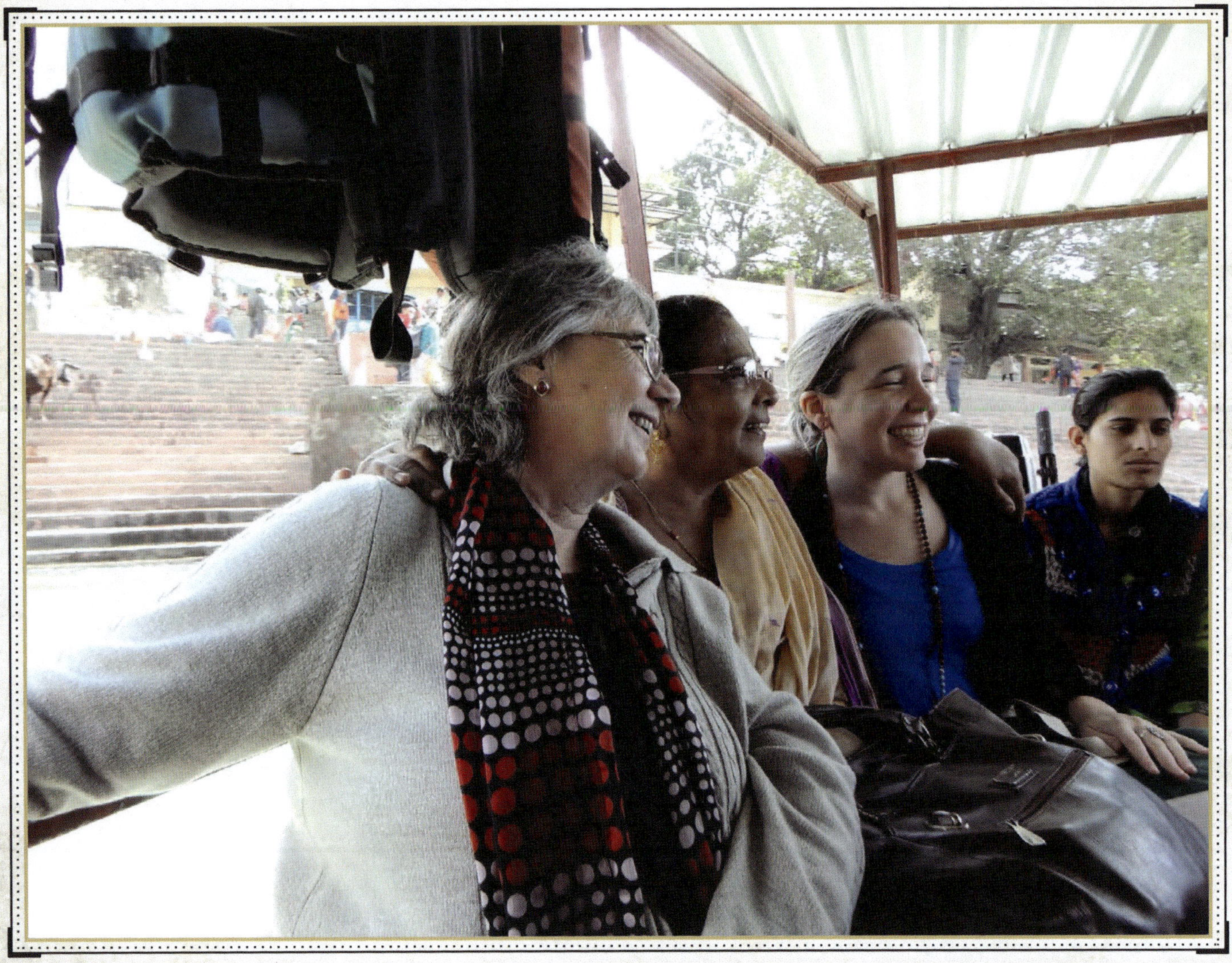

Day 21 and 22

(Rishikesh)

Another disturbing set of dreams of Kelly. In the first, I am visiting a lovely cabin and lake area where Kelly and I had stayed (in my dreams) before. But now I am here alone with only memories. The second dream is where I wake up in my bed alone and know Kelly has chosen not to sleep with me. I go to question him on this and then see he has a huge boil or broken jaw on his right side. I know these dreams are only my own mind churning up disturbances but they make me feel lonelier than ever. I feel Kelly strongly at times and break down in tears of loneliness for his gentle and funny companionship. He had such a wonderful sense of humor and smile and could always laugh me out of serious moods. I still wish him love wherever he is, every night, and make a cup of coffee for him, every morning, along with my own.

Two days in the hotel for me as I have to get this cold settled or I will suffer on my two long flights home. Not helping is the incredible dust particulate in the air that the locals are used to but, as usual, I react to. I am rebuilding my psychic and physical energy. Briefly, I wonder how well I can travel alone after this. It was okay on my first trip to India on a spiritual pilgrimage because Kelly was always there to call and give me support from home. And on the second trip, Kelly was with me and said India was his best long-distance trip out of all of our international trips. I know, though, that I am fully supported when I come to visit India because of my excellent travel professionals who organize all the details of transport and suggestions of places to visit. I tend to check out my own hotels because I know what resonates with me in terms of location and "vibe". In India, English is widely spoken which makes travelling here easier also. All of my support people are fully fluent in English.

Spiritual India always calls me back home. India is not a country so much as it is spiritual energy split into a prism of many colours. I soak in its energy and nourish my soul. I hope I will be back many more times and learn more about myself each time.

My Heart is Left in Shambles

I tried today to meditate

By the powerful and graceful Goddess Ganga

At first it was good

A peaceful mind and gentle feelings

And then you appeared again inside my heart

The one who made me whole

The one who fulfilled my dreams

The one who loved me like no other

The water of the Goddess Ganga could not compare to

The water of my tears

Flowing down my face

And only the chanting priests beside me

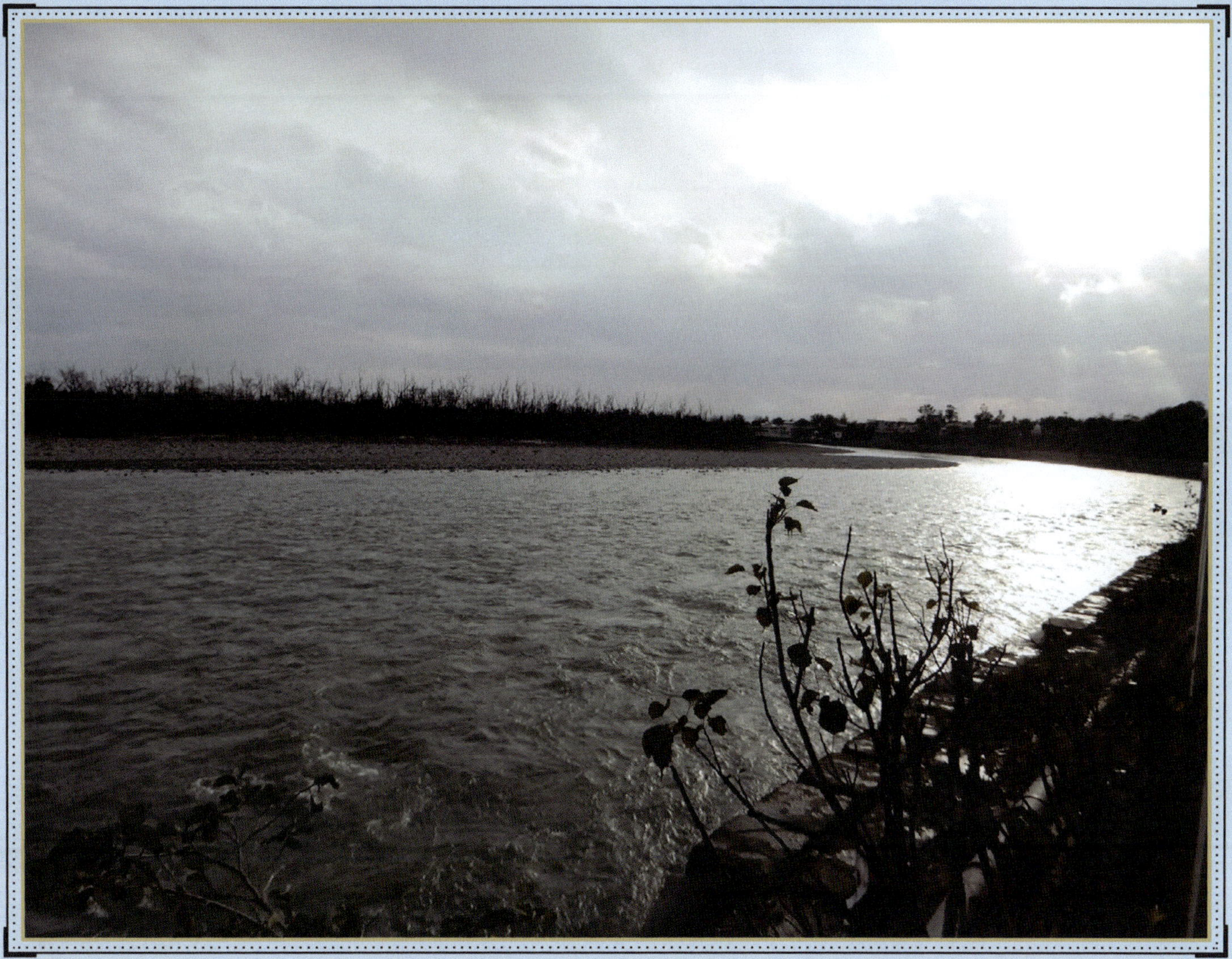

Day 23

(Rishikesh)

A lovely day crossing the Ram Jhula bridge. At first, Santosh and I walk over to the chai shop at the far end and he again orders lemon with ginger and honey. I am still recovering from some sort of cold or dust particulate in my lungs. I read "Autobiography of a Yogi" for about an hour and Santosh reads the newspaper as we sit outside. Then we saunter back to the ashram for lunch for Santosh as I am still not too hungry, although I did have an excellent breakfast. Following lunch, we sit again at the water's edge of the Ganga where the Aarti is performed in the evenings. I sit on a lower step directly facing the huge and beautiful statue of Shiva. Santosh stays sitting above me about ten steps to stay more out of the wind and also to give me a bit of private time. I read a bit and then proceed to meditate but tears and thoughts of Kelly keep coming. I had come to India with some thought of healing the great loss in my heart. I am like a Canadian swan that has lost their forever mate. Now my mate has flown away, and yet, in reality, how many times did he appear to me after his death to show me he was well, excited and healed from physical pain and childhood family trauma. I resolve to focus more on the positive than the negative in the future.

Day 24

(Rishikesh)

As it always is at the end of my journeys, my days start to slip one into the other and I am writing this in the late afternoon of the following day. So begins my recollection of yesterday. I move from the Natraj Hotel to the Aloha on the Ganges. The Aloha was my original hotel but I had come five days earlier to Rishikesh and they had no available rooms for those days. As I near to the hotel lobby, there stands my Vedic astrologer Bhaskar! It is a miracle really as I did not know how to get in touch with him after meeting him in Haridwar. He had said that he could meet me in Rishikesh but the time flew by with me taking two days off and, ultimately, I had decided it would not work and yet here he is! It is a happy coincidence that he is teaching Vedic astrology at this hotel. So, after check- in, I have my Vedic astrology chart done with Bhaskar Yogi as we sit in the spacious and comfortable hotel lobby.

The reading: "I have feet of iron, so although life throws many things at me, I am a strong and stabilizing force in the lives of others, being the iron rods that stabilize the building. Once I was born, things became increasingly good for my family. I do not care much about the making of money knowing that what I spend on others, will come back to me threefold. I will live like a queen until my dying breath. I will begin writing books that others will benefit from. This journal will be published by year's end (five years late – sorry Bhaskar!) and will be of great help to others since it focuses on the state of being a widow from my own fresh experience. I must travel and teach. Bhaskar says I do not usually get grumpy but when I do get grumpy (he is very polite), I should recite "Om Namah Shivaya". He says that although my external life is like a queen, inside I sometimes churn with extra energy and I should recite the mantra to clear my mind. As well, as soon as the mood comes upon me, I should just recognize and acknowledge it, and try to go back to serenity as soon as possible. He says that I had a loss of my father a bit too soon (My dear father was 75 but could have lived longer and my tears well up thinking of the sacred bond he and I shared.) I must be careful not to rush into things as I continue to age, just take my time. My Vedic sign is Pisces with Jupiter as my ruling planet. (In Western astrology, my house of friendship foreshadows these lovely spiritual friends such as Bhaskar and my friend Santosh, as well as many other spiritual friends.)"

The message as a whole is to keep travelling and learning and to share my experiences. To keep knowledge to yourself and not share is like a sin, Bhaskar says. I admit that I have shut down since Kelly has gone away, like I am in a dark cave with no candle. Although outwardly happy, inside I am vulnerable and lost now with regard to direction. Bhaskar has reiterated that although my Venus would want me to take it easy and always enjoy life, my birth Full Moon opposite to my Sun will keep me forever busy. As a final part of this excellent reading, Bhaskar tells me to place water in a clear glass jar and to look at every full moon through it. Kelly and I always used to dance together under a full moon in our lane on our forested acreage with giant Douglas fir trees looking down on us as we twirled.

The reading has a profound good effect on me. I will practise meditation using "Om Namah Shivaya" and also practise visualizing a clear crystal in my 3rd eye area. In reciting mantras, it is an acknowledgement that invisible forces are with us at all times. It is a tough, but normal stage I am going through according to Bhaskar. God appears in a myriad of ways. Kelly is now happy; it is the dredging of my own dark emotions that is what this journal is helping me with. Last night was the first night that I thought that I should take off my wedding and engagement rings just so that Kelly could feel truly released. I thought about it but no, I remembered some time ago in a moment of pique, I had taken them off once near the end of Kelly's illness and he promptly went down to Whoville, retrieved them and placed them again upon my ring finger. So, on they will stay.

It has been a good visit to India. I needed this time in this beautiful spiritual country to clear my mind. I am stuck with my circumstance. Tonight, while resting, I felt someone tap my finger which quickly woke me up. The spirit will come when required. No need to run around looking. My complete focus when I return will be to my cats, Jake and Pekoe, and Fred my dog. I am actually looking forward to just settling for awhile with "nowhere to go, and nothing to do" as an old yoga teacher always opened her classes with.

Today, we visit a very ancient Shiva temple deep in the woods on a mountain top outside of Rishikesh. The monkeys are up to a bit of monkey business as they jump down to swipe the candy prasad but none are so naughty as the Vrindivan monkey from my 2017 India trip who gently stole my glasses right off my nose within a millisecond; he was on a store rooftop before I even knew my glasses were gone. But he was amenable to a trade with fruit by the local grocer and so I got my glasses back and in good shape.

This Shiva temple has a more ornate and elaborate design. As the original oceans were churned and created, Shiva took poison out of the water. His throat turned blue, so here, we pour refreshing and healing water and honey over the Linga to help his throat. One small inner sanctum has a blaze in the middle of the floor with the fire among tall sticks in a metal container representing the destructive power of Shiva.

I had not planned to do anything but sit at the Darshan Ashram but this morning, the wind was too intense. Shiva invited me here instead. If your heart is calm, life will come to you. No need to stress and run here and there. Once I am back at the hotel, I pull back the curtains and see the Goddess Ganga flowing downstream, hear the local Aarti, and see the lush mountainside.

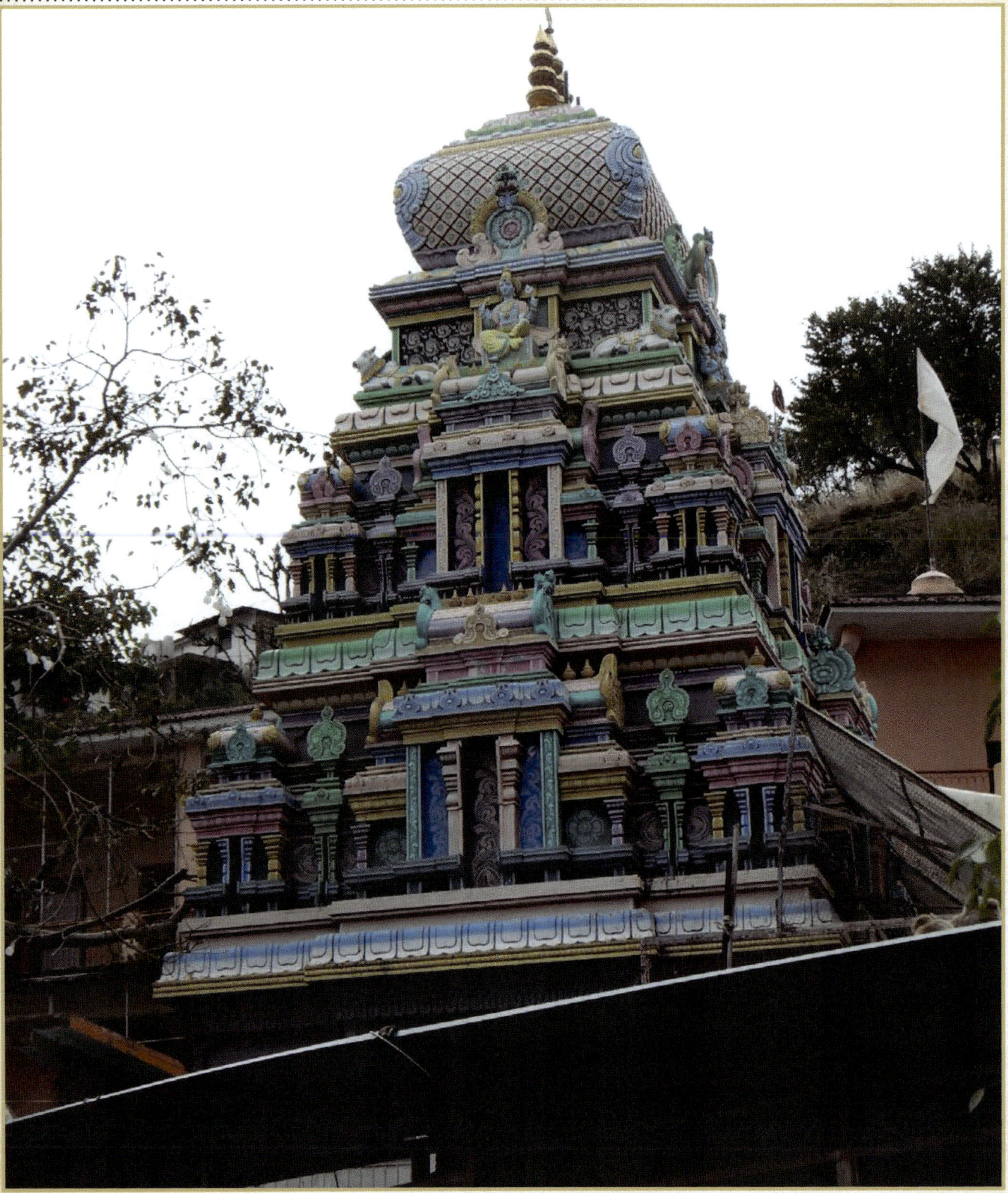

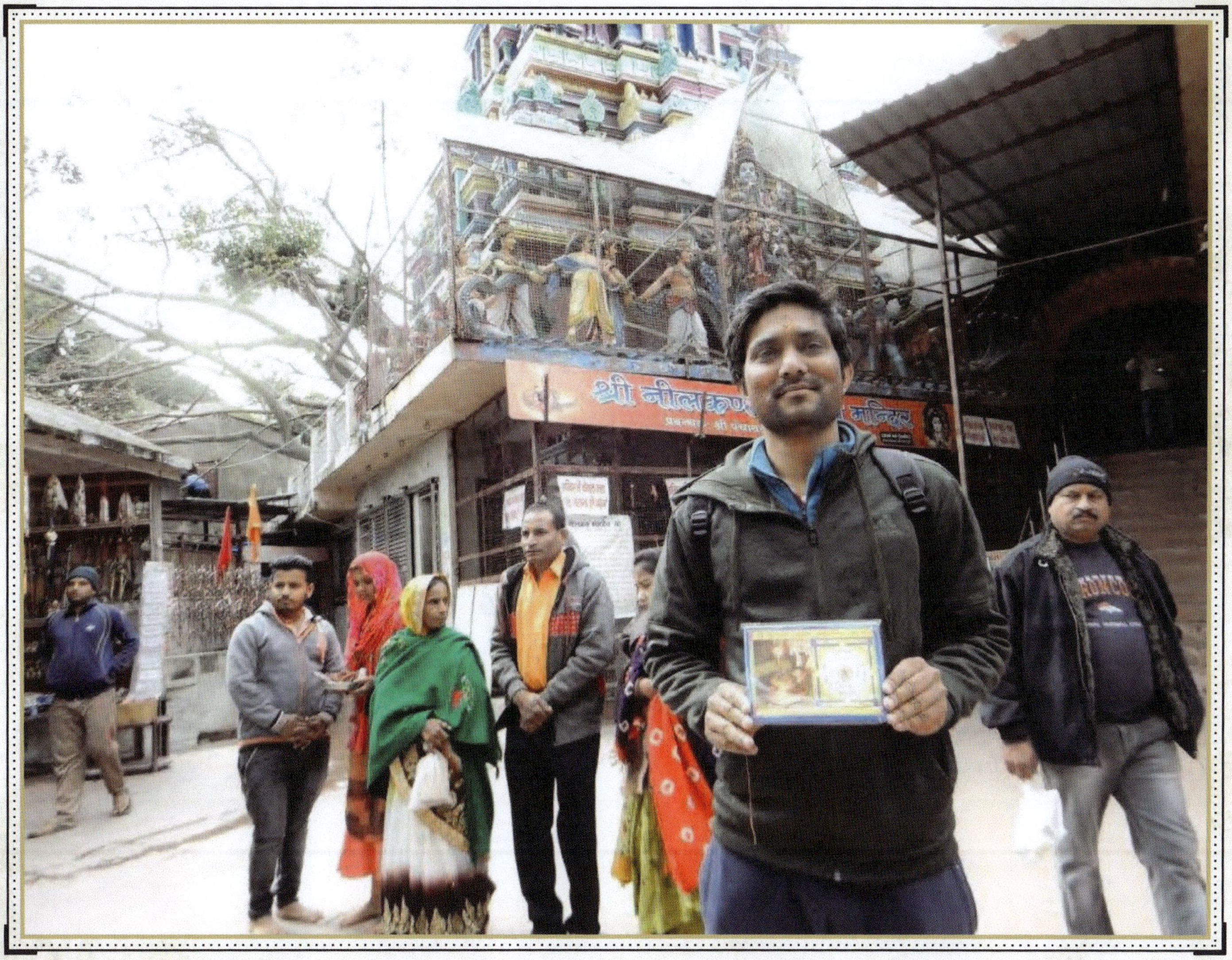

Day 25

(Rishikesh)

Today, I relax in my room except for a stroll to the patio restaurant on the terrace overlooking the Ganges. It is so hot as to be summertime. I indulge in lemon coriander soup and a glass of watermelon juice and a glass of orange juice. I am still reading "Autobiography of a Yogi" and find the parallel of being in India while reading it deepening the experience of the book. This trip is basically over. I am planning for the homeward bound flights. I have no regrets. It has been a time of deep introspection. I have found that I am lonely now without my husband to talk to after the day is done. However, I am so glad that I challenged myself to come back to beautiful spiritual India and especially to the Land of the Gods, Uttarakhand. Now I can just settle in when I get home.

Although the fire in my heart seems like it has gone out, this trip has nourished me and taught me that the world is still full of adventure and new knowledge. I will live a good life based on general survival intelligence and a gracious personality, but I am still healing. My sense of completeness has been shattered. All those who would say, let go, be independent, don't understand that I am by nature independent and free willed. I was living on my own for several years ahead of marriage to Kelly in my early twenties. We complemented each other, and made each other whole – like two sides of a heart that connect to make the perfect union. I am deeply grateful for my amazing life with my husband. He said he would show me a life like no other and he did. He was so capable. He could problem solve all situations and I had perfect faith in him.

Day 26

(Rishikesh)

In the Duncan news a few years ago, I read of a devoted husband whose wife was merely standing at an intersection when she was struck by a car and then died shortly after from her injuries. The obit picture showed a caring and loving woman in her early 60's with her arms folded protectively around her gentle and loved husband. In a heartbeat, his world came crashing down. He says he has left her clothes and makeup exactly as if she is coming home. He is frozen to his spot. No-one should dare to tell him to do otherwise. I keep Kelly's shirts hanging in my bedroom clothes closet exactly as I always have through forty years. One of his Indian shirts, tropical green, is in my suitcase right now. I don't want him to ever think he has been forgotten. I keep my sorrow carefully under wraps in public. But, in private, even the mere casting of my mind in his direction launches a movie screen of memories of everything I have had with his sweet soul shining next to mine.

At the end of this trip to India, I feel no conclusion, only a deep and lonely loss for which there is no repair. My greatest companion is gone, inhaling four deep breaths, and then no more, his death taken of his own powerful accord to release himself from that dreadful late- stage rattling breathing. Even then, he was in perfect control, final breaths and a single tear coming down from the right side of his right eye. He knew he was taking his last breath. He had both a blessed and a cursed sixty-five years because his early life was made harsh by negligent parents, but through sheer will-power, he educated himself, gained a high-end technical trade, married well, travelled around the world, biked, kayaked, lived on a sailboat for ten years, and took five acres of wild forest and created an estate with hand-hewn stone pathways and a small town affectionately called "Whoville". After all of that, it came down to this single shocking moment. I am so grateful but forever scarred, as only those who have gone through this can understand, at that quintessential moment, the instant moment of the complete summation, the little boy having to face his greatest fear in that winter sun-lit room with the door partially open to hear the wind in the trees. I leaped immediately to hold him after I heard the sudden change of breath and knew what happened.

My brave soul, my little boy who only wanted fun and joy. Just know the joy you gave to others is beyond measure. You made so many people happy. You created so much good will, good works and harmony. I thank God that I met you and you shared your life with me. At the end of the day and at the end of this journal, I am honoring you and saying to you, you lived a worthwhile and noble life.

I sat with you once the doctor had come and gone. I sat with you and held your hands, rubbing them constantly, constantly leaning over to kiss you. Your face had a joyous look, a warmth, an indescribable glow, one of peace and contentment, like you had licked your final foe. I sat with you for five hours, just the two of us in the house we had built together, just like we had planned, nothing to take us away from each other. At the first, your mouth was open and I tried to use a handkerchief in Irish style to close it – I was sure you were laughing hysterically from above. I gave up and left the room briefly and when I returned, even though you were technically dead, you had closed your jaw! I do not doubt in miracles, my husband, you are the master of power and self-control. I sat for five hours holding your hand, absorbing your glow and my profound loss at that incalculable intersection. And then I got tired and having been given a two-hour notification request by the funeral parlour, I called to say that "pick-up of the body" should be in two hours. How was I to know you could hear me? When I returned to you, your face was hard and cold and even though your eyes were closed, I could see you looking upwards to the skies, filled with the purpose of leaving this world truly behind. My husband, at that point, you were truly gone to me as my life partner in this physical world.

And then a few days later, I was alone at the crematorium watching the smoke stack billowing the white smoke of your atoms into the sunny but cold air. I took your ashes home warm knowing that your spirit had risen high above earth, and I poured your ashes along with your old friend dog Charley's ashes, exactly where you used to sit in the stream exalting in all the natural elements.

My love, you came with the gift thereafter, of speaking to me three times to let me know you are happy and eager in your new life. A disembodied voice right beside the bed on your side. You can imagine how shocked I was but also exalting in the joy of your continued life. And you came in profound spiritual readings. I understand that you now stand and receive lonely souls coming over who have no family and friends to meet them. And there you are, with them looking at you and wondering who you are.

I am sure that with your beautiful smile and joyous laughter that they now know they are home.

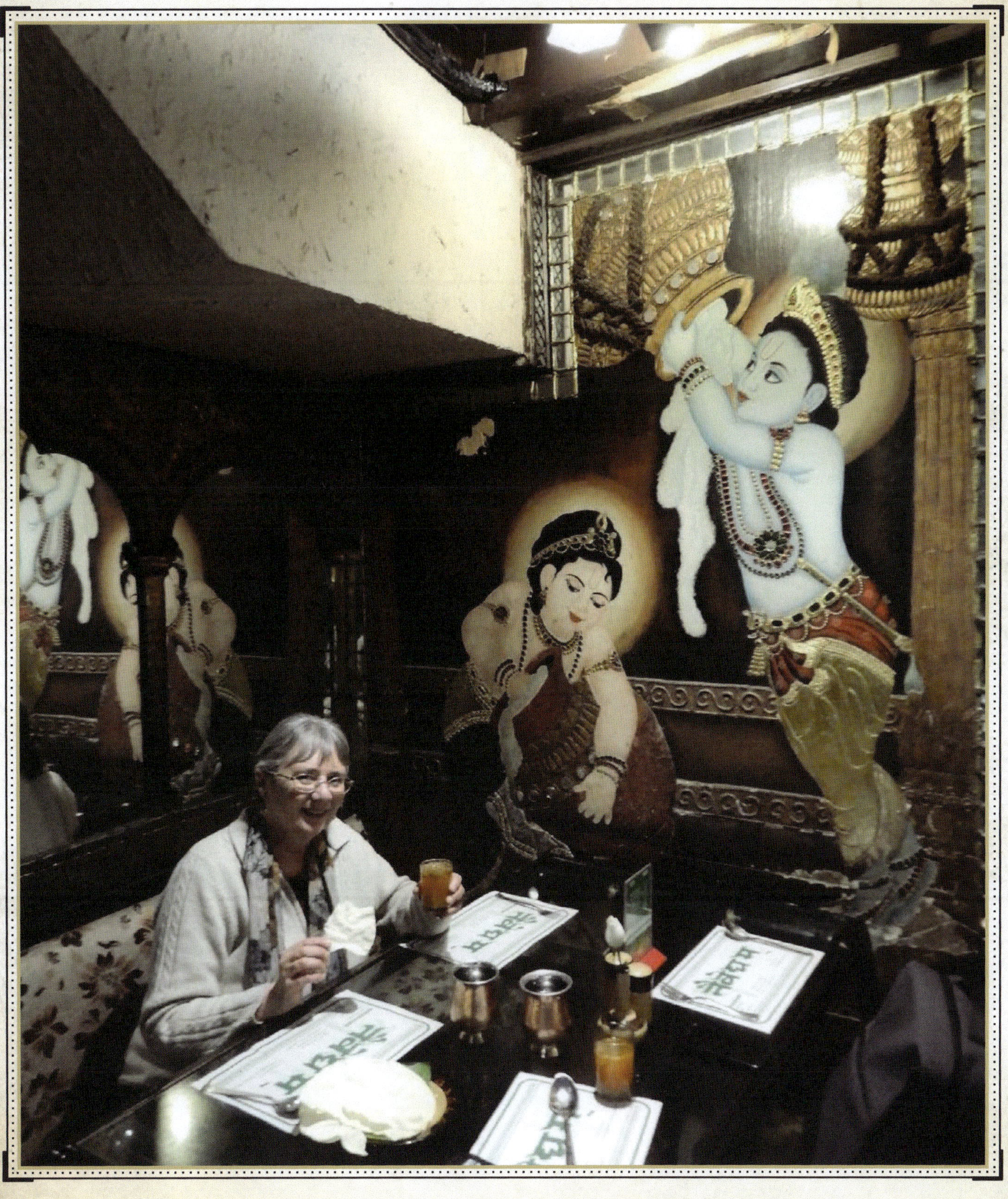

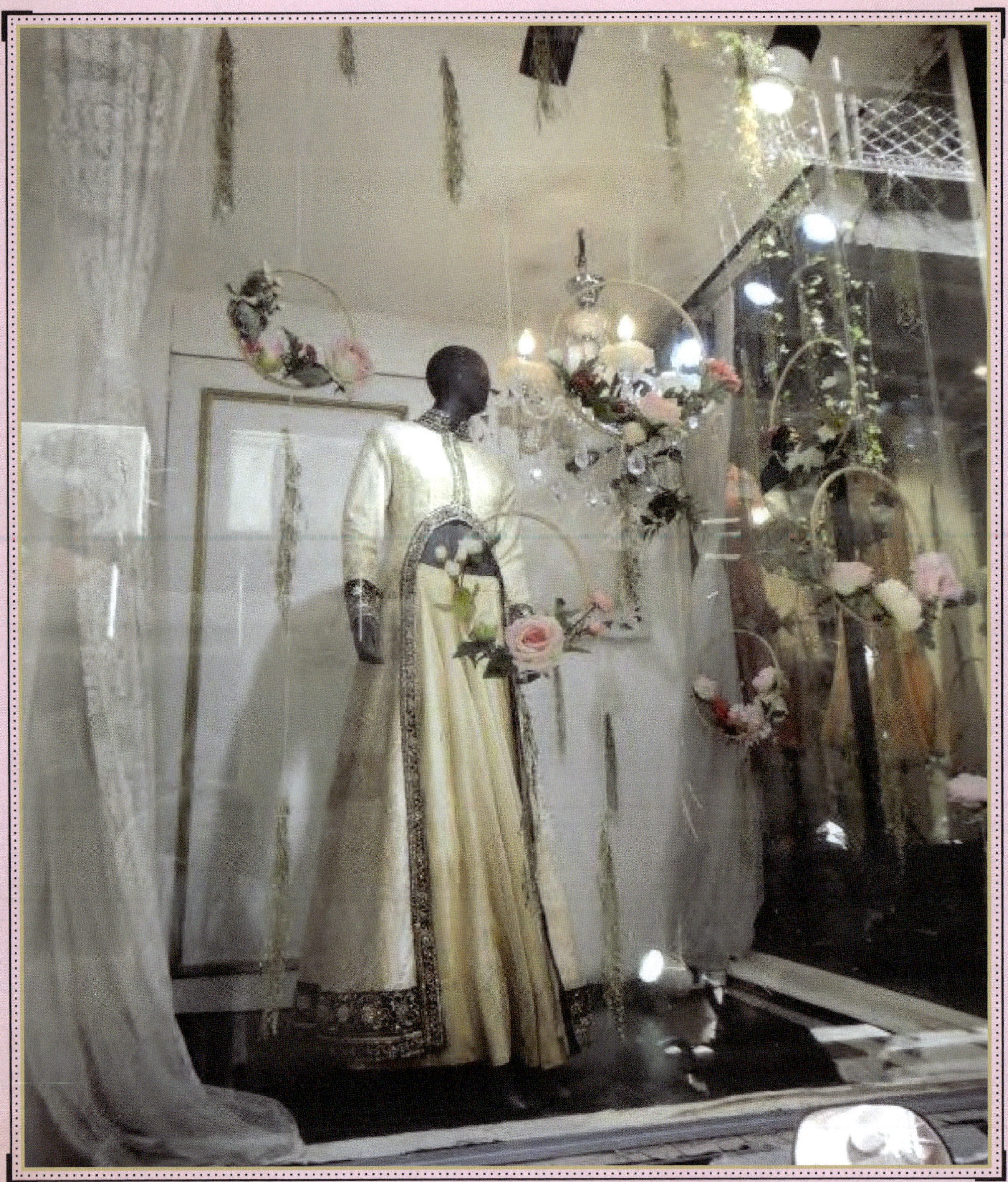

Epilogue
Five Years Later

Even five years later, I still feel my husband over my shoulder, an invisible presence of support and love. I will never forget our last conversation, the day before he died. "I love you so much, there are no words."

He was ever the poet with a voice I wish with all my heart that I may hear again. From a drawer, I have randomly pulled out a handful of yellow sticky notes, large enough for small ditties. I began hearing these small poems in my mind, even as soon as a day after Kelly was gone. In his life, he would often suddenly come up with lyrics, none of which he wrote down; it was just a natural talent. And now I can suddenly hear complete little sets of words and I write them down. Somehow, he passed that on to me.

Nothing changes, I still love you with all my heart, And wish we weren't apart.

I did my best to love you well, And the results only time will tell.

It is set in gold your love for me, Like molten lava hardened in the sea.

His delicate touch is indelibly in my soul scribbling notes, encouraging me to laugh. Like two streams, we met to make a river, and then went side by side again. We may yet meet again in the great cosmos and mystery of life. But it may surprise you to know that I am now fully engaged in life. Creativity, joy, the love of friends, colour, gratitude, and enjoyment of the single moment bless me constantly. I am embracing this late stage of life for my remaining time on this spinning miracle called earth.

Two years after Kelly's passing, one morning after I woke up and lay in bed for awhile, I fully embraced the complete quietness of his non-self, the emptiness of the room, the lack of heartbeat next to me. I faced it full on. I listened intently to the absolute silence surrounding me. At that point, I had the choice to wither but instead found the strength to know that Kelly is in the next heavenly room living his own life and that I need to embrace my own life with joy and heart. Time and space are an illusion; how many sages have said that. I need only to think of Kelly and he is there in front of me, loving me and encouraging me to keep going. There is so much more to learn while I still have the breath; and even after the last one, I will continue to embrace the mysteries of the universe but in a different form. I am sure that Kelly will be dancing an Irish jig to meet me and he will say with a twinkle in his eye "so darling, what's our next adventure?"

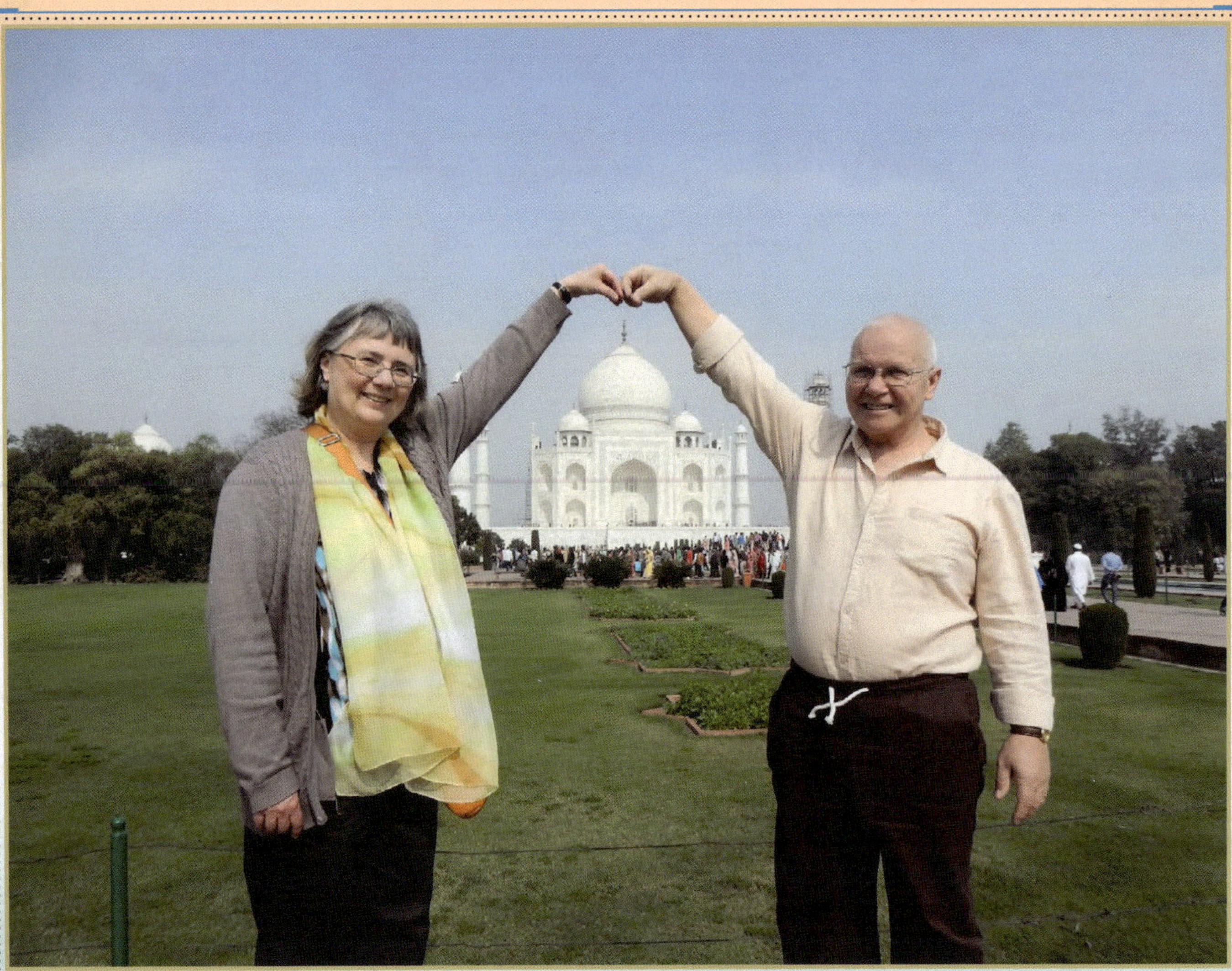

Kelly and I at the Taj Mahal, India in 2017.
Another dream come true for two adventurers who came together in life, in love.

I AM TRULY THANKFUL

Writing this book has been cathartic. It needed to be done. I needed to thank my husband and feel that his soul is shining brighter in the starry heavens because of the love I am sending to him with these words. Grief does not need to be endless although it feels like that for many years. Many good friends pulled me up at that time and made me stronger. I would like to mention especially having the anchor of three special decades-long friends. I have known dear friend Sharon since I was three years old. We have aged together and she is one of my pillars of identity. And my dear friend Linda, who was my maid of honour at my Lutheran church wedding, wrote a letter to Kelly every few weeks of his two-year illness. It made him feel special at a time when he couldn't believe that his world was literally collapsing. And dear friend Liz always called with an infectious joy that made the whole house light up. For someone who is going through trauma, a simple letter or phone call means the world to them.

Kelly had two amazing friends, Paul and Maurice who, in the saddest of events, had both lost their wives to cancer in the previous year. Feeling they needed to do something to revitalize themselves, they embarked on an adventurous motorcycle trip through Mexico and Central America. They made it a point to visit Kelly on our property before they began their big journey. It meant so much to Kelly to have them by his side as he showed them his creative work of stone pathways, hand-hewn village called "Whoville", and stained-glass work. We followed Paul and Maurice in real time, as they posted their adventure online. It gave Kelly a break from always thinking about his own situation. I have the deepest gratitude for Paul, and also for my special friend, Darlene, who both went out of their way to help me in my darkest hours after Kelly passed, with phone calls and visits. If you are suffering, call on friends; some can help, some may not be able to, but reaching out is really important. Hospice Care Centers have grief support groups and people who can come to visit. They know not to intrude; you are in control of your own grief process.

For myself, after having worked through all the paperwork, pension adjustments, selling my home and moving to a completely different area, I really needed to do something, like Really Big to get myself on track again. So, I decided to go to India. For me, India is my second home. A place where I can rest my soul. It is exciting, the food is delicious, the people are considerate and generous, the culture is bright and full of hope and yet also full of an ancient sweetness that I have never found anywhere else in the world. You can easily travel to India as a solo woman if you have found yourself a good travel professional and for me that was Mr. Praveen Juyal with Whoopee Holidays India. He arranged all the details of my extensive itineraries including travel guide, car and driver for each of my three trips. My travel guide has always been Mr. Santosh Sharma. Santosh and Kelly hit it off from day one of our 2017 trip. Kelly loved history and Santosh was thoroughly knowledgeable of the architecture and cultural importance of every place we visited. I also appreciated an amazing hotel manager, Mr. Jaspal Bisht of a Delhi Justa hotel, the first hotel from my first trip to India. His attention to detail, friendliness and complete professionalism gave me that initial feeling of wanting to come back again to India.

India nourishes me spiritually. Immersing myself in temples where the rooms are closed while the Gods and Goddesses are bathed and given lunch is a very strange concept for the Western mind but it is completely harmonious to the Indian concept of feeling divinity as an everyday reality. The invisible world is very visible in India. A strong spiritual belief gives me infinite comfort. My meetings with my Naadi astrologer in Delhi, Mr. Thanapal Kanagaraj, and my Vedic astrologer in Haridwar, Mr. Bhaskar Yogi, have been life changing in understanding the subtle dimensions and incorporating those understandings into my own daily life. The Om symbol on the first and last pages of this book represents the sound of the sacred essence pulling all variables into unity. My deep Christian roots are in complete harmony with the loving spirit of India. Learning to understand the purity of my own soul is an on-going personal project. This book would not be complete without thanking the Reverend Patricia Gunn, Church Minister and Founder of the Cowichan Spiritualist Church of Healing and Light, for her amazing spiritual readings that have lightened my heart and opened up my soul to those higher realms of existence. I can only aspire to her level of cognizance.

You can survive the loss of that special someone whom you have built your life around, trusted and depended on. Working through grief is knowing that you have a bit more time left, and that you can open a door to new experiences if you want. I try to plan two big projects every year now. This year, it is writing this book and then finishing an astrology certificate course from Oxford, England. Next year, it will be completing a dragon cross-stitch as it will be the Year of the Dragon, my husband's sign, and secondly, reading the Bhagavad-Gita in its entirety. So, it is step-by-step now in enjoying my creativity and maintaining good friendships, gardening and photography. As well, a whole new world of writing is opening up. I have so many journals of places that Kelly and I travelled to – Cambodia, Vietnam, India, South Africa, China, and many local kayak and canoe experiences that I have written down over the years. I am going to share these journals, as well as spirituality, photography and poetry on www.phoebewriting.com which will link to e-book platforms. I would love for you to come along! Just like me, it is a work in progress!

There is more to writing a book than putting evocative words in type. The beauty of "A Widow's Journey to the Land of the Gods" comes from the absolute artistry of my amazing graphic artist, Ms. Nicola North. After each e-mail to her, and there were many, I always ended with "Namaste, and thank you!" Nicola's take on every illustrated page continuously astounded and delighted me throughout our collaboration. I am ever so grateful for her expertise in bringing the words of this book into illumination. As well, I am so lucky to have found First Choice Books in Victoria, British Columbia, to bind and print my book. I have dealt with them before and they are meticulous in the process of book publication, as well as being local.

In one of my special spiritual readings after Kelly's passing, he came through to say that "over there" is a beautiful large library building in which is contained the first edition of every book ever written. When it is my time, I fully intend to have an armful of my published books to carry over for Kelly to place in that dome of knowledge. I look forward to mingling and sharing ideas. I hope they have cookies and coffee!

My last words go to Kelly - when we came together, everything became good.

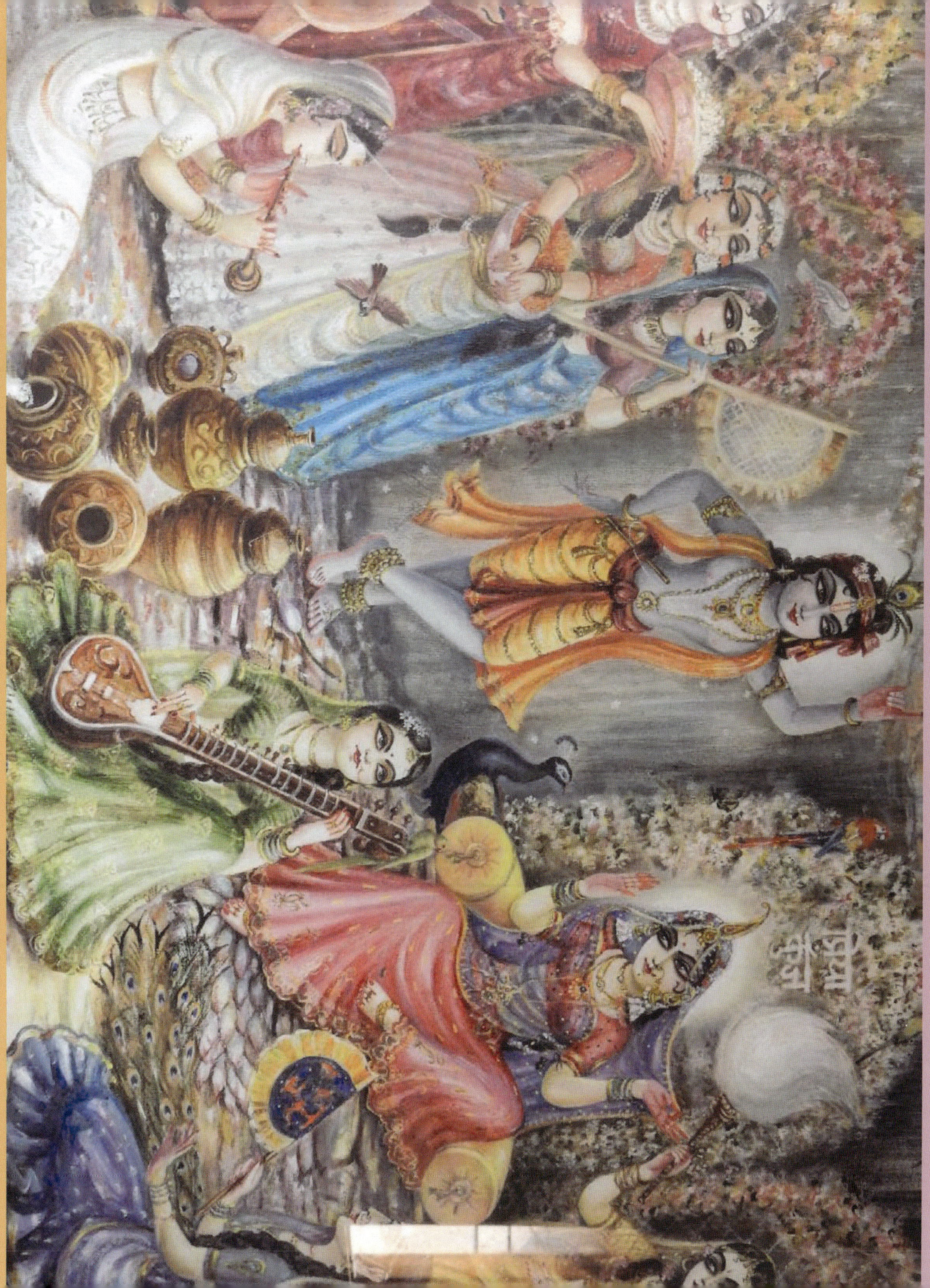

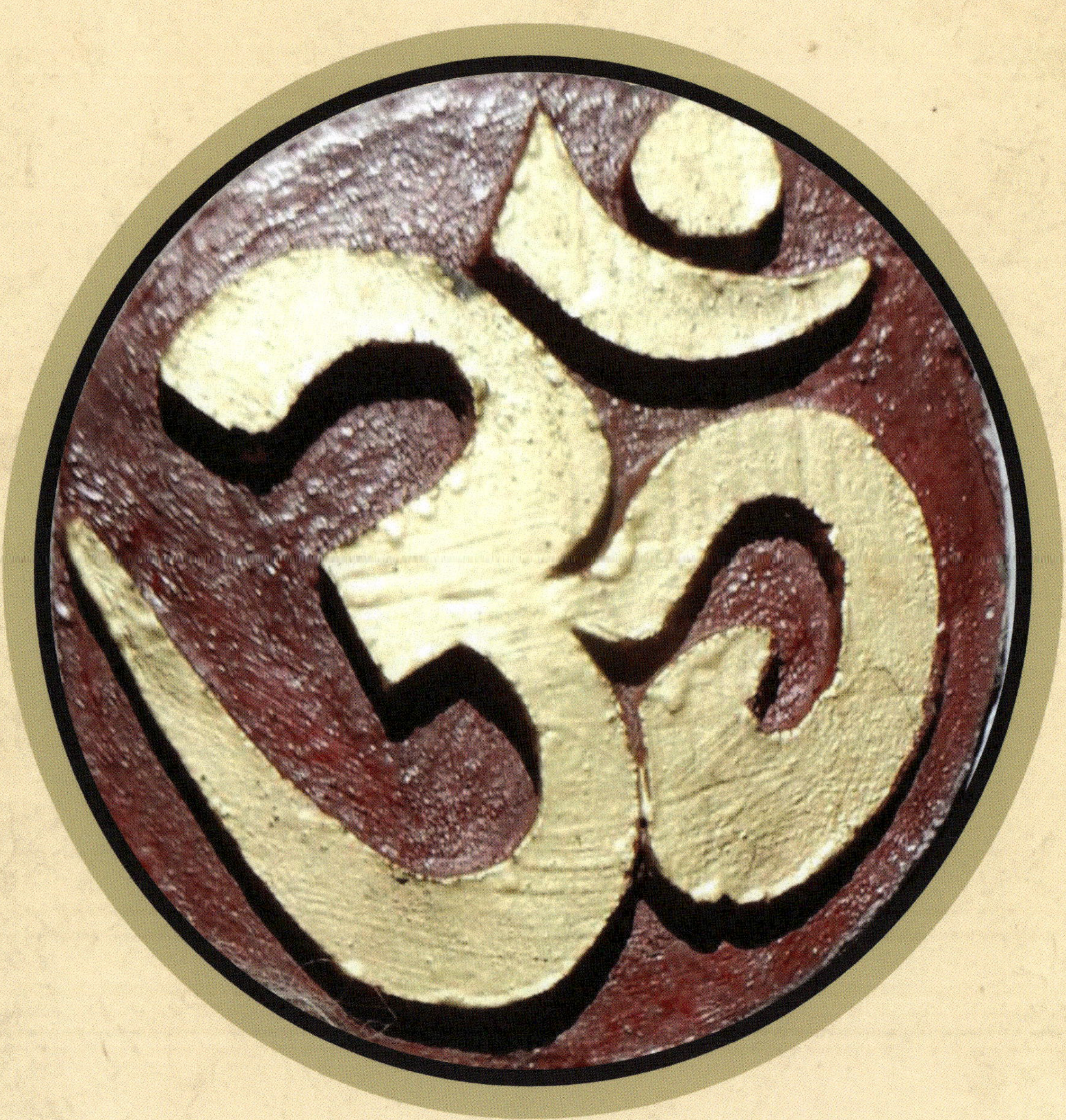

Printed in Great Britain
by Amazon

30257437R00064